The Men on My Couch

The Men on My Couch

TRUE STORIES OF SEX, LOVE, AND PSYCHOTHERAPY

Dr. Brandy Engler with David Rensin

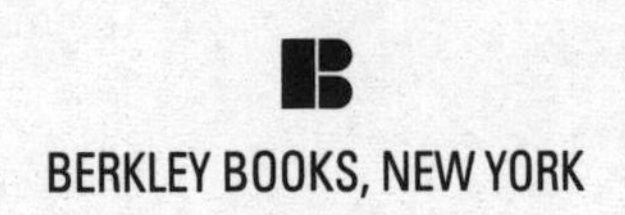

BERKLEY BOOKS, NEW YORK

THE BERKLEY PUBLISHING GROUP
Published by the Penguin Group
Penguin Group (USA) Inc.
375 Hudson Street, New York, New York 10014, USA
Penguin Group (Canada), 90 Eglinton Avenue East, Suite 700, Toronto, Ontario M4P 2Y3, Canada (a division of Pearson Penguin Canada Inc.) • Penguin Books Ltd., 80 Strand, London WC2R 0RL, England • Penguin Ireland, 25 St. Stephen's Green, Dublin 2, Ireland (a division of Penguin Books Ltd.) • Penguin Group (Australia), 707 Collins Street, Melbourne, Victoria 3008, Australia (a division of Pearson Australia Group Pty. Ltd.) • Penguin Books India Pvt. Ltd., 11 Community Centre, Panchsheel Park, New Delhi—110 017, India • Penguin Group (NZ), 67 Apollo Drive, Rosedale, Auckland 0632, New Zealand (a division of Pearson New Zealand Ltd.) • Penguin Books, Rosebank Office Park, 181 Jan Smuts Avenue, Parktown North 2193, South Africa • Penguin China, B7 Jaiming Center, 27 East Third Ring Road North, Chaoyang District, Beijing 100020, China

Penguin Books Ltd., Registered Offices: 80 Strand, London WC2R 0RL, England

This book describes the real experiences of real people. The author has disguised the identities of some, and in some instances created composite characters, but none of these changes has affected the truthfulness and accuracy of the events described.

This book is an original publication of The Berkley Publishing Group.

THE MEN ON MY COUCH

Cover design by Diana Kolsky.
Cover photo: Man on Couch © Bernicce / Shutterstock.
Book design by Laura K. Corless.

PUBLISHING HISTORY
Berkley trade paperback edition / January 2013

ISBN: 978-0-425-25334-2

An application to register this book has been submitted to the Library of Congress.

PRINTED IN THE UNITED STATES OF AMERICA

10 9 8 7 6 5 4

The patients' names and all identifying information have been changed and in several cases are composites in order to protect their rights to confidentiality. The dialogues and events are all based on actual conversations and experiences, although some have been weaved together to create a singular case. I have also changed the names of my friends and love interests.

CONTENTS

INTAKE

The Men on My Couch is the story of my unexpected journey into the erotic minds of men. What I learned there, about my patients' desires and behaviors at the intersection of sex and love, not only took me by surprise, but challenged my assumptions about both men and myself.

There are many ways a woman can explore the truths about love and herself. Some go to meditation centers or take a solo journey into the wilderness. Some purchase a pile of self-help books, venture into online dating, or train for a marathon. Others take off for a wild weekend in Vegas.

I just had to go to my office.

A few years ago, as a newly minted clinical psychologist, I set out to fulfill my dream of a private practice in Manhattan. I had just one small obstacle: I wasn't established yet. Anyone in my field will tell you that building a clientele takes time. Several colleagues suggested that I should take the slower, more conventional route: join an existing group practice, get involved in the community, and network with medical doctors, college psych departments, and other professionals who could generate referrals. I considered their advice and the financial benefits of taking a job, but I had just completed specialized training in sex therapy with a renowned practitioner and was brimming with enthusiasm. My supervisor at the Brooklyn hospital where I had just completed my residency warned against the idea. "Sex therapy? Are you kidding me?" he said. "That's outdated. Everyone's on Viagra now. Nobody gets sex therapy clients anymore."

He offered me a position at the hospital, but my mind was made up. I hung my shingle in the heart of Times Square. I didn't care about Viagra. I had written my dissertation on low sexual desire in women and I wanted to specialize in female sexuality.

I expected that building my clientele would be slow. I'd learned during my research that while women are more likely than men to get therapy if they suffer from anxiety, depression, grief, etc., they rarely seek help for low libido because they tragically assume that their waning passion is normal. So slow was fine with me, as long as I was doing what I wanted to do. And with this issue being so pervasive, I thought that if I advertised my services, the women would eventually come.

I was wrong.

The calls began immediately.

And almost all of them were from men.

Men? Not quite what I had expected. And within a few months, I had more of them than I could manage. They called with all kinds of sexual concerns: chronic womanizing, porn addiction, prostitutes, sexual identity issues, jealousy, erectile dysfunction, fear of intimacy, loss of desire, trying to understand the meaning of love, and more. Men may be less likely than women to seek psychotherapy for many of their emotional ailments, but when the penis doesn't work, they reach out.

Even though treating men for sexual issues was not the type of therapy I'd set out to do—although, of course, my training had included that—I thought I could help, and I sparked to the challenge. I suspected that I was about to hear stories that might unsettle me, but like the bold but naïve horror movie heroine who's compelled to figure out what's going on despite suspecting that the killer might be lingering in the shadows, I was curious. So I summoned a bring-it-on attitude, opened my office door, and started taking appointments, ready to face whatever adventure awaited.

I wasn't disappointed.

The Men on My Couch will take you inside my confidential therapeutic sessions to witness powerful and provocative dialogues that reveal the core issues underlying male sexual behavior. From a fly-on-the-wall perspective, you will observe the raw emotions and actual motivations behind the modern sexual maladies for which my patients sought help. And unlike most other books about male sexual behavior, in *The Men on My Couch* you'll also be privy to my professional *and* personal reactions, both those shared in the sessions and those that remained unspoken.

I soon discovered one constant truth: Sex is rarely just sex. Sex is a loaded experience. Although at the outset I thought I'd be treating sexual symptoms, most everything quickly boiled down to the psychology that drove my patients' behavior. I began to uncover all kinds of meanings attached to their sexual habits. Some employed sex to act out suppressed emotions or to mollify uncontrollable emotions. Sometimes they sought to reexperience and master old traumas that lay deeply embedded in their fantasies. Many used sex to meet frustrated needs for power, approval, self-worth, comfort, and affection. Usually, my patients had limited insight into the motivations that drove them. They instinctively sought healing on the sexual playing field, and the results were often dysfunction and disconnection.

I'm not going to pretend that I have all the answers about men, or that I can tell women how to change the men in their lives in order to have a wonderful relationship. Nor is this book a polemic meant to suggest that men whose behaviors and attitudes don't conform to whatever passes for our socio-sexual mores are bad. I do, however, take a hard look at men in this book, often challenging them to the point of their anger and tears. And yet I do so with deep regard for them and for my privileged position as their confessor. Thus it is important to me to avoid the pejorative and facile portrayal of men as superficial and morally flawed scoundrels—you know, dogs, pigs, incorrigible bastards—even though at times these thoughts crossed my mind. I am not trying to excuse or justify their behavior. I am not asking you to take pity on them, or even to forgive them for damage they may have caused you; rather, I ask you to witness this journey of insight into the psychosexual motivations of men—and what they discovered in the process.

Instead of telling you what men think or want, I will let you read what they told me. I offer my analyses and my personal reactions to the men, not just as a psychologist, but as a woman. *The Men on My Couch* is not simply a series of case studies, but my own journey of development and discovery, a diary of the lessons learned in the therapy room and how they impacted my romantic relationship. When I opened my practice, I was involved in a tumultuous long-distance relationship, and just like my clients, I was caught between my desire to love and not really knowing what loving meant. When it came to romance and sex, I had for a long time dwelled largely in a wonderful, self-created fantasy world where my lover and I could hold hands and perpetually skip through the sunny fields of enchantment. When I fell for my boyfriend Rami (not his real name), "love" took on different qualities. Love was suddenly raw, volatile, and unpredictable. We had hot sex. We had trust issues. We were from very different worlds. A passionate tug-of-war ensued, and I was often on the losing end— and not without fault.

As I went through that relationship, the lessons I learned were heightened and informed by my work. After all, how many women are in their daily professional lives also in the business of exploring the reefs and shallows of love and sex from a man's point of view? How many hear truths *about men from men*, truths to which they have never been so forcefully exposed, much less imagined?

At first, this combustible information cocktail threatened to explode in my face. Some sessions left me dazed by revelations that quickly became questions and suspicions that I would inevitably apply to my relationship with Rami.

Fortunately, I eventually realized that I could make my work with men *work for me*, and I began to develop a new understanding of love. As part of the process, I had to confront many of the assumptions that I, and many other women, hold about men, and discover that they were often far from true. They include: "If he loves me, he won't cheat," and "If I'm thin or pretty or seductive, or play by certain rules, he'll always want me."

For example, a close girlfriend once told me, "I don't think my boyfriend would cheat on me. He just seems like he's so into me. He does everything for me. He cleans my car, he cooks my dinner. He doesn't have a super-high sex drive or seem that sexually adventurous. He just seems really happy to be with me."

I hope she was right. But as some of the patients in this book demonstrate, being in love with a woman does not guarantee sexual fidelity. Nor does unfaithfulness imply that a man's love is inauthentic and that he doesn't take it seriously.

One common assumption is that men just want sex—and maybe a pizza and a beer afterward. And then they want sex again. I can't tell you how many times I've heard a girlfriend complain, "He just wants sex." And yes, men would come into my office just talking about sex. "I'm not getting enough," or "I can't get it up," or "I like oral sex and she doesn't."

But they'd inevitably wind up talking about love.

The truth, I learned, is that men *do* want sex, but not *just* sex. Listening to my patients, I realized how strongly *a need for deeper connection* lay beneath the sexual behavior—a need that was often difficult to communicate to the women in their lives. From there it was a short step to better serving my patients by exploring the content of their hearts, rather than condemning what their penises had done.

The Men on My Couch is not clinical. It's not self-help. There are no lists, exercises, or affirmations. It trusts you to read the stories and, taking from them what you want, make up your own mind. We all know too well that there are no pat answers about love. This book, then, is an exploration. My purpose is to take readers on the journey with me, in vivo, as I was learning myself. My hope is that this book will provide a new perspective on sexual and relationship dynamics, an alternative to readers—particularly women—because when I talk with my girlfriends about these subjects, we *always* get around to wanting to know what men really want, wanting to understand why they behave the way they do and what we can do about it.

Finally, although all the men in this book are different, they share a common thread: They're not perverts or deviants; they are everyday guys, from all parts of the country and a variety of social strata, who could be anyone's boyfriend, husband, brother, or friend.

They are the men we all know, and the men women want to know about.

DAVID

David was a young, rising star in the financial world. He had a girlfriend who modeled professionally and an apartment in trendy Tribeca. He carried himself with a self-assured ease and the courtly grace and charm of a young man from polite Charleston, South Carolina, society, raised to be a gentleman. Tall and lean, with a solid football player's body, he wore an expensive suit and walked into my office with the commanding presence of someone who knew what he wanted and was used to getting it. His eyes swept the softly lit room and checked out the wall art with an approving glance before casually focusing his appraising gaze on me.

"Wow, Doc. You're pretty attractive," he said. "I think I'm going to like talking to you."

I blushed. I felt a bit flattered by a handsome man's compliment, and also a bit intimidated, which alerted me to what was likely happening: He wanted to sexualize me in order to establish a position of power. He was one of my very first clients, but I was sanguine about his comment. I had been well prepared in my training for dealing with patient projections, and I wanted to focus on getting beneath his polished persona. His opening line let me know that he had to be masking some level of discomfort about the naturally vulnerable position of patient, especially one speaking to a woman his age about sexual matters.

I gave him a warm yet professional smile. “I’m glad you feel comfortable around *attractive* women,” I said, reflecting back his word. I gestured at the couch. “Have a seat.”

David sank back into the cushions and ran his hand over the sleek black leather. Pelvis forward, legs open, arms spread, he ran his gaze up my legs and body. I met his eyes when they locked on to mine. This was obviously going to be a chess match. He had opened with a nuanced offensive, and the challenge of breaching his defenses intrigued me.

Despite his provocations, I actually didn’t find him to be very enticing. His eyes had a dull, vapid look that betrayed a lack of authentic charisma. His charm seemed scripted, and his magazine-cover face was almost a turnoff because of its proximity to perfection. Yes, great looks will get a woman’s attention, but in the end she wants to be the pretty one.

David settled in and I asked him what he wanted to talk about. I half-expected another flirtatious riposte. Instead, he went in the opposite direction. “I don’t know if I’m capable of love,” he said, softly. “I don’t think I even know what love is. What is love, really? Can you help me?”

David’s inquiry seemed earnest and sincere, and he looked at me expectantly. I paused, caught slightly off guard, and realized that I didn't have a ready answer to this simple yet difficult question. What is love?

Sometimes I think patients assume that psychologists are the keepers of the secrets to life's existential quandaries: What happens when we die? Do soul mates exist? Is there a God? But that's not the case. We observe human behavior, prod, listen, reflect, and try to lead our patients toward finding whatever conclusions work for them. To explain the meaning of life, and in this case love, is better left to spiritual teachers, biologists, and philosophers, who will happily provide their theories and dictates.

So I decided to meet his search for an answer with a question. I simply asked David to expound on his interest in the discovery of love.

"My girlfriend is absolutely gorgeous," he explained. "She's tall and blond, a model with a perfect rack and rock-hard abs. I don't know why, but I cheat on her. I can't stop myself. She works at night and I go out with the guys for drinks and right away we start collecting numbers."

As a young woman and neophyte therapist, I experienced a sharp and unsettling visceral reaction that jolted my stomach and raced up through my chest. Sitting in front of me, reaching out for my help, was the embodiment of any woman's worst fear: the proud philanderer and skilled seducer who womanizes insatiably with complete indifference to his committed relationship. I was immediately contemptuous and had to hide it behind my well-rehearsed therapy façade of nonjudgmental neutrality.

"Collecting?"

"Yes. There's a process to it," he said, rewarming the cocky charm, "and I am known for being the best. First, I scan the bar for the hottest chick and make small talk. I try to make a specific compliment about her beauty while remaining underwhelmed. I know how to be aggressive without seeming eager. I want to appear to be truly interested in who she is, so I ask questions without talking too much about myself—except for occasional references to my financial status. I let her talk about herself and I listen for what she wants and I make that what I appear to have to offer."

I don't know what was more abhorrent about his actions: that he could not be satisfied no matter how perfect the woman in his life was, or that men share a secret knowledge about how to manipulate women and use it for group sport.

David rearranged himself on the couch while I imagined that scenario. "Then, I do the 'Take Away,'" he said. "I turn as if I have lost interest, or I start to show interest in another girl—but never one of her friends; that's an amateur mistake. I let her work to get my attention again. If she doesn't, I will still talk to her, but I've moved on. Either way, my attitude is casual yet interested. Works every time."

"Okay, how often do you do this?"

"Several women a night maybe."

"And the object is to . . . ?"

"Collect phone numbers. Maybe more. It's exciting, like winning a game," he said.

I scribbled a note to explore his competitive nature. "So you follow through and have sex with these women?"

"Sometimes. But never more than once."

I could see him brace slightly for possible approbation. Instead, I took an encouraging and even approving tone. I smiled and nodded along as if I was totally nonreactive to what he was saying, as if his story was just like all the others, another routine day in the office for me. It's a tactic I often find useful in getting the patient to tell me everything. "How is the sex?"

"Pretty good," he said, relaxing a bit. "But I mostly like the process of going to the bar with the guys and getting the numbers. I'm more interested in the hunt than having sex."

David's description had shown me which phase of the womanizing process was most important to him. The apex of this type of interaction can be different among men. I believed that exploring the most favored part of David's pickup experience would reveal the clues to what issues really drove him. For example, some men are happy just to be able to look at women. Some get off on meeting them. Some men want sex, and others require the women to fall in love with them. David's thrill was obtaining a phone number. Even though he sometimes slept with these women, an invitation to follow through if he desired was all he really needed.

David's story reminded me of how one of my girlfriends had complained to me that a guy she'd been dating never complimented her and at times flirted with her friends. "I can't figure out if he's really into me or not," she said. Then one day she discovered a book in his bedroom called *The Game*. She flipped through the pages, horrified, then bought a copy of the book for herself and showed it to me. The book was a collection of techniques for seducing women taught by a supposed master pickup artist, and apparently there was even an online community for readers to exchange advice.

Together we felt like we'd unearthed some mystical—and evil—underworld of male machinations. Everything this guy my friend was dating, and David, had been doing was straight from this nefarious pickup protocol: ignore her, refrain from compliments, or give a compliment then negate it, like . . . "I like that you're pretty, but not model pretty." This scheme basically taught men how to get into a position of control over the interaction by trying to evoke insecurity and, by questioning what she has to offer, trying to get the woman into the role of selling herself to him.

The rational part of my brain realized that these techniques could work short-term, but long-term they would only engage a woman's ego, and the strategy would eventually backfire. Still, it was upsetting to know that some men treated "relationships" as just a game. My girlfriend decided to eavesdrop on the online "community" and was so insulted by what she had read that she decided to post the following: "Hey nerds, Dungeons and Dragons called, and they want their players back!" We laughed at her little jab, but did she break it off with her boyfriend? No.

I felt contemptuous of David and his like-minded manipulators. Yet I couldn't act on that feeling with some snarky comment or walk away like I would have had I met him in bar. I'm a therapist. I'm supposed to help. I knew that good therapy is supposed to utilize empathy, but I didn't feel any.

I realized that I needed to control my countertransference—the jargon word for my personal reaction. A therapist has to be mindful about which of her personal issues are provoked so that she doesn't respond to the patient's issues with her own issues. In other words, in sessions I have to be aware of what's their stuff and what's my stuff, because all therapists have stuff that can be unearthed by the patient. Like all therapists, I have to know the difference and monitor that constantly.

I used our remaining time to give David the sexual status exam, the first-session standard assessment tool that provides a snapshot, or more like a movie, of the patient's most recent sexual encounter. I wanted to know who initiated, what kind of foreplay occurred, what positions, the amount of eye contact, and what thoughts and emotions he'd experienced. I also asked about masturbation practices and the specific content of fantasy.

I discovered that so much information about a man's personality and emotional needs can be extrapolated from his sexual behavior. I can get a sense of his ability to love, self-esteem, level of assertiveness, personal power, and even issues stemming from childhood. Sex is a microcosm of the self.

Initially, asking such questions made me a little embarrassed. I was even a little uncomfortable with being called a "sex therapist," a title that to me had always conjured images of old ladies fascinated with sex toys. I had chosen to study sexuality from a very analytic perspective, and thanks to my conservative upbringing, I could still easily blush over the graphic candor needed for sexual discussion. For example, I found myself avoiding the word "fuck," and instead would say "making love." This wasn't because I was uncomfortable with my own sexuality; really, I'd just been brought up with Southern decorum and etiquette. We speak in polite euphemisms. My mom always reminded me of the importance of being "ladylike" and that I came from a lineage of very proper and pious women, the kind who wore long dresses and pearls do to the dishes.

After David left, my tentative assessment was that despite his bravado, his responses were loaded with self-consciousness, fears, and competitive tendencies. The obstacle for me in treating David's style of relating was that it had become part of his identity, and once a patient's pathology becomes an important part of his identity, he has a hard time making any real changes. I deemed my chances at building insight in David low, but I did see one possible opening. The womanizing, usually a source of pride, wasn't quite enough anymore. He was aware that he wanted to experience love, he just wasn't sure what it was. I wanted to help guide him there, so I had to pause and reflect on my own relationship with love.

I thought, at the time, that I knew love very well. Love was romance, of course. In fact, I pretty much had an ongoing, grand love affair with love. I had loved men, yes, but my true loyalty was to love itself. I had over the years, developed an ability to cultivate the euphoria of romance. It's a skill that I honed, and I had been successful at drawing men to me, not because of my looks or my intelligence, but because they wanted to feel intoxicated by it, too. I could create the sensation of love at any time with just about anyone. And once in that state, it was easy for me to believe that no man would ever have malevolent intentions toward me, because I semiconsciously projected a certain innocence that tended to elicit a man's protective and nurturing instincts. David and I in the room together were sort of like Don Juan meets Pollyanna.

The next time I saw David I went back to his unanswered question.

"So," I said, "You wonder if you're capable of love . . . ?"

"I guess."

"Have you thought any more about why?"

"Maybe it's because I sabotage every relationship by cheating with women I don't want to become attached to, women I could never fall in love with. Is that strange?"

"Do you think it's strange?"

"What's strange is that even though I don't care about them, I still compare them to my girlfriend."

"Sexually?"

"Not really. I imagine a life with each of them."

I didn't expect that response, and David anticipated my next question.

"I really want to settle down and get married. I'm financially stable now, and all of my friends are getting married and buying big houses in Westchester and Jersey. . . . I just want the hottest chick and I want the biggest house."

Between sessions I'd thought a bit about David's competitive nature. Since he said he wasn't necessarily turned on by the women whose numbers he collected—guys aren't always aroused and can even be turned off by women they pursue—I suspected that his nights out, scoring phone numbers with his friends, were less about the women and more about the gamesmanship. In other words, his womanizing was socially driven, in terms of his relationship to other men.

David confirmed my instinct when he told me that he'd come from a high-achieving, performance-oriented family with several brothers, the kind of environment that creates either anxious perfectionists or those who eventually collapse into depression from the pressure. David was driven. He'd quarterbacked his high school football team. Now he ran a successful hedge fund with the same aggressive and strategic thinking. He worked marathon Wall Street eighty-hour weeks. I knew men in that business. Some blew off steam by using cocaine and Russian hookers. David didn't seem the type, but I needed to check.

"I don't like to pay for sex," he said. "I just like to pursue hard-to-get women." But when they sparked to his interest, David lacked the empathy, or social intelligence, to be aware of what his "prey" might themselves be feeling: the excitement of meeting a handsome, well-to-do guy; the enticement of a good prospect, possibly marriage material; hoping that he was interested, and possibly feeling some anxiety caused by an acute awareness of the lopsided ratio of women to men in the city. I wanted to give David some insight into how the women he hunted might feel. I wanted him to trade places with them. I moved my chair closer and leaned in to emphasize our connection. "What if a woman you're talking to is feigning authentic interest in *you*?" I suggested.

David smirked, openly skeptical.

"What if she only sees you as a *giant dollar sign* and is scheming ways to manipulate you into taking her shopping or traveling? What if the entire interaction at the bar is fake with *both* of you playing a part?"

David quietly considered my suggestions, and I watched as the answer slowly dawned in his expression.

Insecurity.

He'd never considered that a woman who acted interested in him might not legitimately want him. He needed to be desired, and if he sensed that desire from a woman, it *couldn't* be fake. His ego counted on that.

"It's important to you that the woman *truly* desire you," I said, gently explaining what he now seemed to realize, but had previously not thought about.

David's body language began to shift. His cheeks pinked as anxiety and shame rose to the surface. He drew one arm across his chest, raising his hand to his chin. His brow furrowed, his foot tapped in a staccato beat. I watched his ego deflate in slow motion. The nightly escapades that had once had such powerful value for him were suddenly infected with doubt. I had created a rupture in his ego and for a moment I felt hopeful that now we could start to do some real therapy.

I adjusted my position in the chair and looked at the floor for a moment to ease the pressure. When I focused on David again, I could see a flash of defeat cross over his face. Aha. Checkmate. Yet I didn't feel victorious. The air in the room was heavy with a new presence: emotion—his and mine. I felt a warm wave of compassion well up inside of me. Neither of us spoke for a long moment. This was the first time I'd felt empathy for David.

"What's happening inside you right now?" I asked softly, feeling a bit vulnerable myself.

"Nothing," he snapped. "I need to go. I have a meeting in thirty minutes." David jumped up abruptly. The room went cold. I watched him walk out of the office. I knew I should have tried to keep him in the room, but it had all happened so fast, and I felt hurt. I had made a mistake. I had been trained that when a client wants to leave early, that's a classic sign that he's running away from something and that it's crucial to address it right in the moment. I wasn't sure if he'd be back.

Fortunately, David did return the following week. But he arrived twenty minutes late, with no explanation—another classic sign of resistance. I was happy that he'd shown up, but his tardiness likely meant that he wanted to truncate the session to avoid being seen on a deeper level.

Further, David's early cockiness had also resurfaced in full force. As he sank into the couch, he said, "You look nice today, Doc. You know, you *really are* sexy. If I saw you outside this office, I would try to talk to you."

This time I wasn't flattered or offended. David's return to sexualizing behavior was transparent. He'd eroticized his anxiety and retreated into his safety zone of power-seeking objectification. This wasn't unusual: David obviously felt exposed and that explained the reversion. Now I was back at square one with him.

I didn't want to be sexualized. I've only ever wanted my patients' respect. And their approval. I wanted my interpretations and techniques to be taken as clever and astute, wise and helpful. In fact, I felt a rush of confidence each time a patient would say "That's exactly it!" or "My life has changed for the better!"

And yet I knew that aspects of my physical presentation could be taken as seductive. The fitted skirts, the high heels, the crossing and uncrossing of my legs, the attentive eyes or the soft therapist voice. Once, in grad school, a male supervisor had pulled me into his office and advised me not to wear tall boots with skirts to the office because I might distract my male patients. (Meaning I distracted him?) However much I may have enjoyed the attention on a subconscious level, I didn't abide his advice. My clothes were perfectly reasonable. I was dressed like every other young professional woman in Manhattan that I saw on the streets each day. I didn't want to wear formless dresses or boxy business suits. I wasn't trying to be provocative, just fashionable.

My physical presentation didn't become sexualized until I walked into the room with my clients. So I decided that if the men on my couch were reacting to my physical presentation—assuming my grad school supervisor was correct—then this meant opportunity. Their sexual and emotional issues would rise to the surface, and then we'd get to deal with them in the moment. In other words, I used their reactions as a tool to help them understand the way they related to women.

The way a patient acts in session is usually a mirror of how he generally interacts socially. It's called *transference* when the patient projects his habitual relationship patterns on to the therapist, who then reflects them back in order to help him. Although it's not unusual for a sexual current to flow for a variety of reasons, from the innocent to the chemical, David's attention to my body and his easy flattery suggested that erotic transference was a pattern for him. This really wasn't about my boots.

I have often become a symbol for the women in my patient's lives; or more accurately, the beliefs that they've developed about women. They may be projecting issues with their lovers: the aloof woman, the rejecting woman, the nurturing mother, the critical mother, the seductress. Some idealize me and others devalue me; their reactions to me reveal their deepest wishes and darkest motives as they cast me in a role in their own personal drama. I was vigilant about who my patients thought I was, or needed me to be. Did I represent women who turned them down? Women they couldn't get? Was I an ideal for them? In David's case, did he see me as one of many potential conquests?

I typically address erotic transference immediately, but in this moment, I decided to bypass his flirtations and go for what I sensed would be just beneath his behavior.

"I was concerned after our last session," I said. "You left pretty abruptly."

"Yeah. I had a meeting."

Rather than question his hasty explanation, I stayed on a personal level. "I felt uncomfortable with our last exchange."

"Me, too," David said, his voice flat.

"Can you be specific about what caused your discomfort?"

"I just never thought of it all being an illusion."

"What was most difficult for you about that realization?"

David sped past my question. "I guess I just really get off on having girls want me," he said. I affirmed his bitterness instead of criticizing it.

"So having girls want you is very important to you."

"Yeah. I guess."

"What do think that means about you?"

"Fuck, I don't know. I guess it means that I feel better about myself when I seduce women."

"Is that why you act seductively with me?"

"I find you attractive; what's wrong with that?"

Now it was my turn to deflect his question. "What is it like for you, having this kind of conversation with me?" I kept my voice soft, but held his eyes.

"Uneasy at times. But I can handle it."

"So it seems. You walked in. You told me I was sexy. That's your usual pattern of relating to women. You're confident and seductive . . . and yet," I wore my concerned face, "hard to reach.

I'm having a difficult time actually connecting with you. I wonder if this happens in your relationships."

I'd struck a nerve. "That's true," David said quietly. "My girlfriend, Nikki, complains that I don't open up."

"What do you think she means by that?"

"I don't know. That I'm not capable of love—at least the way she thinks love should be? Isn't that why I came in here?"

"Tell me more about Nikki."

"I think she might be 'The One.'"

"What makes you think that?"

"I know she loves me and I think she'll be loyal to me. And she's hot. That's why I can't understand why I keep hooking up with other women."

What was it with this guy, that he had to continually go there? People who are so wrapped up in how hot they are, how hot their lover is, what kind of car they drive, the size of their house, seem to me lame and immature. I was drifting into being judgmental again, and I couldn't help myself. Such superficialities seemed manufactured and callow. I imagined David and his cronies cruising the bars, roving bands of post-college frat boys in khaki pants—boring, banal, prosaic. But worst was the arrogance and crudeness, the vulgarity of "She has a great rack, rock-hard abs." He wasn't celebrating her physical beauty in this declaration to me; there was no hint of reverence or appreciation in the way he used the word "rack."

My reaction to his language was based not in morality or my Southern prudishness but in the dehumanizing effect. However, I sensed that indignation might have led me to some answers for David.

Although David had *described* Nikki, we hadn't talked about her in much depth. I wanted to know more about how she and David spent time together, about their connection—beyond her loyalty and hotness.

"We hang out with friends," he said. "We go to bars, or stay in and watch movies. Lots of sex, too. She's amazing in bed."

"Yes? What do you like most about sex with Nikki?"

"She really gets into it."

"Meaning?"

"She's uninhibited; she likes it, too," he said, a comment I began to learn was the most popular description of what makes a woman a good lover. "She'll do *anything*," he added with a seductive grin and extended eye contact.

David was flirting with me again. His tone invited me to ask just what "anything" meant. I refused to give him the satisfaction. He told me anyway. "She screams, she writhes, she has multiple orgasms."

"That's wonderful," I said.

"And I can tell she isn't doing it just to make me happy," he added, a touch defensively. I guess my earlier suggestion that David should try to imagine a woman being dishonest must have struck a chord. "I'm pretty good at what I do. She makes me feel good and I know that she wants me. Do you want to know more?"

Not really. I wanted, sadistically, to pop his bubble of grandiosity. I actually wanted to club it, like a piñata. But I knew that that was not the way to build a therapeutic relationship with any patient, especially one with narcissistic proclivities. He had no ability to see the true value in a woman, and by this I felt offended, and rightfully so; this trend of dehumanization is at the heart of all sexual harm. In fact, I wanted to fight against it, not with a club, but by helping David. I intended to use my relationship with him to create for him a new and different emotional experience of a woman.

To get David to open up to more authentic feelings I had to align myself with his narcissism. Trying to ram up against the blustery defenses of a narcissist only increases the swagger. Instead, I had to mirror back to David those qualities he so fancied in himself, show him that I got why he was so fantastic. That's the trick to getting a narcissist to respect you. This was hard because I was forced to acknowledge a truth about David that I preferred not to see. He challenged the fantasy image I wanted to hold of men: that they are equally obsessed with Victorian-style courtship. He was popping my romantic bubble with his boorish words that felt like ransacking Barbarian invaders, reducing my high ideals to vulgarities. He saw women as prey. If he could have stuffed and mounted on his wall the women he took home from bars, he probably would have.

In truth, David appreciating Nikki's hotness *wasn't* about her at all. It was one-sided. He'd made a statement about himself. Her physical measurements represented something about *his* self-image. Her "writhing, screaming, and multiple orgasms" let him know that *he* was a good lover, that *he* had caused her pleasure, and that *he* was therefore desirable. Feeling good about oneself is fine, but the equation didn't seem to include Nikki at all. She was simply a sexually stimulated and vocally appreciative audience in a play about David. This was the work of ego—in my view, the great disconnector.

And herein lies the precarious balance between self and other in all human relationships. Imagine a continuum, where on one end your romantic partner is treated as an object to service all of your needs—sort of like the relationship between a mother and a baby. At the other, you are able to recognize your lover as an actual person with needs of his or her own and ideally there's a balance of give and take.

It seemed to me that David spent his time on the object end, focused on how to get validation and keep it coming. He felt exultant or sad, entitled or worthless, always in some state of reaction to the need for obtaining affirmation and what he thought was love. For him, the act of *giving* was for women, Mother Teresa types and fools. I began to notice that many people implicitly hold these expectations. If stated outright, however, they seem pretty outrageous. I tried to imagine what this would look like in the form of a contract given at the beginning of a relationship. It would go like this:

> *I want you to do what I want, when I want it. I want you to be what I want all the time. In fact, you are an extension of me. I want you to give me what I need exactly when I need it. I shouldn't have to ask for it or tell you how to do it. I want you to give me love unconditionally. Guaranteed. Unrelenting. I want you to be my savior, my Jesus, my mommy or daddy. And if you don't, I will be pissed off! I might even leave you or cheat on you, because my needs should be met at all times.*
>
> *P.S. I don't want to hear about your needs.*

Now imagine introducing yourself with that on the first date. Relating to people as objects is at the core of narcissism, a phenomenon so harmful to relationships that I should take a moment to explain further. Even though the term "narcissism" gets thrown around about a lot of deserving or not so deserving men—even I use it for convenience—I don't actually like it as a broad label for individuals, as if only a pathological few of us exhibit this tendency. Narcissism is a state of mind, a distorted way of viewing the world, a particular type of myopia through which the world is processed in a kaleidoscope of personal expectations, beliefs, and yearnings—none of which are based in objective reality. In the most pervasive and maybe most damaging form, the afflicted wear blinders that block their ability to see others except in terms of themselves and what they want. This is harmful because without the ability to see others, we begin to objectify one another.

We all do this to some degree, and it's pretty much a pestilence on modern relationships. It's the opposite of self-love; it's being trapped inside one's self.

David not only couldn't see others, he had to be *better* than them, too. Narcissism in this fashion is a sense of self constructed around a need to be special or superior to others. Everyone is viewed in terms of hierarchy. Others are either beneath you or above you, with constant comparisons calculating in your mind. Dictates like *I must be rich or beautiful or the best at whatever I do* take over. Even if they're high-achieving in reality, this type of narcissist lives in an illusion because the acceptance-seeking that underlies this striving is ironically never gratified; if such narcissists achieve that perceived superiority, then they are actually *separating* themselves from others.

So, yes, we all have a bit of narcissism in our relationships. Even in my own romantic love fantasies I objectified men, but instead of making them sex objects, I made them my love objects.

Part of the problem for David was that when one's ego is aggrandized so easily, as it is for a successful guy like him, the pleasure of the ego-feeding can be so reinforcing that there is no compelling reason to stop. I recognized that David couldn't even appreciate having a relatively satisfying relationship with Nikki. I needed to get him to examine *why* he needed to hunt women nightly.

David's narcissism was a place of power and safety. I had to get inside it. This time with a much softer tone.

"My hope is that you understand that I'm asking tough questions to help you explore yourself," I said the next time we met. We were still talking about Nikki.

"I'm not used to it," he said, his shoulders collapsing. "I feel exposed and I hate it. I'd rather be in control."

"You say that you love Nikki, but what does love actually *feel* like in your body when you're together?"

"I don't know." He sighed. "It's out here somewhere." David grasped the empty space in front of his head. For David, love was an abstract concept with no visceral component. Love was disembodied. I'd encountered this before and the thought alarmed me: Why were people having so much trouble *feeling* love?

"Is it possible that your need to control the relationship and avoid vulnerability blocks your ability to experience love?" I suggested.

"What do you mean? I *love* my girlfriend."

"So you *do* know what love is."

"Well, I . . ."

David could go through the motions of affection with Nikki, but he didn't actually experience the warm, contented well-being of loving. Instead, all he could identify was a hunger for this elusive state.

"I hear that she loves *you*. But in fact what you've described sounds like your need is not to be loved, but to *feel desired*. You want to be wanted, over and over. You can't get enough of having women desire you. But who do *you* desire?"

David had no answer. I kept pushing. "To desire someone requires that you give something of yourself, that you allow yourself to also *feel* love for someone. I don't see you taking that risk—yet. Only when you can tolerate that risk will you have real power."

Silence.

"What are you really chasing? Love or validation? To love someone requires . . . balls."

"You're pissing me off," David said, scowling, wrapping his arms across his body.

"Good. What are you pissed about?"

"I fucking feel fucking embarrassed, shallow and . . . pathetic."

"Great," I said. "You're finally letting me see *you*. Thank you."

"You're welcome, I guess."

"Good. Now we can do some work."

The next time I saw David, he rushed into the office, atypically distressed. His usual cool demeanor had been replaced by panic. No more flirtation or coy small talk.

"I think my girlfriend has been cheating on me," he blurted. "But she denies it."

"How did you come to that conclusion?"

"I looked in her cell phone and found a text message from another guy saying that he was on his way over. The text was sent at three in the morning. She claims it was just a friend and the text was a mistake. I was so pissed. I went home and started going through my phone numbers."

Ah, the phone numbers. David's security blanket. The symbols of his prowess. The keys to prevent him from unraveling.

"I called this hot brunette that I met at Buddha Bar the other night, and she invited me over to her place." His voice dropped to a disgusted whisper. "But when I tried to have sex I couldn't get a fucking erection!"

I frowned sympathetically.

"I kept thinking about Nikki the entire time," he continued. "I couldn't stay focused. Even when this chick went down on me I couldn't stay hard."

David's self-loathing had come to a crisis point, a good opportunity for him to grow. He had tried to deal with his pain by retreating into a night of sex—and he just couldn't escape. Now his defenses had broken down. He felt rejected. He felt like a failure. It was like watching a boy cry because he didn't make the team.

"You're mad at yourself for not getting hard when you had a lot to be upset about?"

"Yes." His chewed at his bottom lip, then retreated into anger. "Fucking bitches."

"You're angry. It also seems like you're hurt and believe that you can't trust women."

"They all cheat," he said in a cold declaration.

"Yet, you *need* women, you need to be loved," I said warmly.

"Yes" he said, his face dropping in a fleeting moment of hurt.

"But you're afraid to trust them," I said, tilting my head, my eyes searching behind the restraint I saw in his clenched jaw.

"I guess that's why I have one and keep lots of backups," he said, retreating into his pattern.

"And that makes you feel safe?"

"Yes. Yes. I just hate to be alone. More than anything. I can't stand it. I get so bored. So I start calling everyone I know looking for any girl to go out with."

"So, not only is being without a relationship scary, but being alone in your apartment, even for one night, is too much."

"It's like I can't be comfortable in my own skin."

"Can you describe what that feels like?"

"I don't know," he said, struggling. David was so disconnected from himself that he was unaware of his own internal experience. But I wasn't about to let him off the hook. This was important: being able to identify something that drove him so powerfully.

"Try and tell me what it feels like in your body."

"I don't know," he repeated. I waited. I could have assuaged his unease by giving him the words, but I had to let him figure it out for himself. Eventually, my silence pressured him into a response.

"I guess it's an . . . emptiness . . . here," he said, pointing to his chest. "And a restless energy. It's a dark moment . . . as if I don't exist. I panic. I have to call a woman. It's an urgent feeling. And I can't tolerate it."

Finally, an honest breakthrough after months of therapy. We had come to the pain that drove his behavior.

"Sounds like a profound discomfort."

"Yes, which is why I go to the bar, or start calling women."

"So, you deal with your fears of being alone, and in this case being cheated on, by getting women to express their desire for you."

"But I don't want to get into a relationship with those women."

"Right. You avoid a deeper connection. These women are like a mirror for you, reflecting back your worth. Without them, you don't exist."

"It's fun sometimes, though."

"I know it's fun and it feels good for you," I said. "You look to a woman to make you feel good about yourself. But then you get let down and fixate on how untrustworthy women are. You let a woman determine if you are lovable or not. What's missing?"

"That I don't feel that on my own."

"That's a lot of power to give to another person. You want confirmation that you're lovable, but even when you get it, it's never quite enough. It seems to me that the result of all this is that while you're trying to gain power, you're actually losing it."

"I never thought of it that way."

I leaned forward to close the distance between us.

"I need to love myself?" he said, almost ready to laugh that this conversation had boiled down to a therapeutic cliché.

"Yes. That is your ticket out of this pattern. If you can find love from the inside, you don't have to keep chasing it from the outside."

"All right, Doc. All right, I trust you."

David thought highly of himself, but he knew that I could deflate him very easily. He had to stop building his self-worth based solely on the external reinforcement that he got from his career, his physical appearance, his financial worth, the messages he got from his family and lovers, etc. They were not sustainable. His looks would fade, finances fluctuate, and women fail him. There was no constancy. In order to feel worthwhile, he would need to learn to provide validation for himself. He would need to begin to accept and appreciate himself and allow a process of self-exploration.

"How does one get started?" he asked.

"You need to let go of what everyone else thinks and find yourself," I said. "You need to honor what intrinsically motivates you—even if you don't know what that is right now. It may be exactly what you're doing, but you'll have to be willing to start over without the women and find out."

Though David's narcissism was pernicious, it was really an attempt at self-acceptance. He'd been seeking the safer, less vulnerable alternative to real love, but I was pushing him right into his real fears so that he couldn't avoid them anymore. I thought that if he could confront those fears with me, it would help him to get ready for love.

After work, I strolled through the muggy summer evening, down a street lined with restaurants and cafes and up to one of my favorite spots for thinking, an old sofa chair on the rooftop of my apartment building where I would sit and look out over what I pretended to be my living room—Manhattan. It was relaxing to watch the commotion of the city from a few stories up, and it provided me a removed perspective, both from the chaos of the city and from my own emotions, so that I could reflect more on David. I was arriving at a sense of peace about our work, with no more need to beat him like a piñata; I felt like he was truly open to change.

He had reached an important place. He thought womanizing made him feel better, but he'd finally realized that it made him feel worse. But self-love is no easy task, particularly in the face of the powerful reinforcement David got from his career success, peer and parental approval, a model girlfriend as an ornament of social status, and the ability to seduce other beautiful women to repeatedly demonstrate his worth to himself. This striving to prove himself to others was a powerful compulsion that had disconnected David from who he might really be and masked the emptiness he felt when he was alone.

During the next few months, David began the slow process of self-exploration. He was introduced to an alternative social circle through some artistically inclined friends who spent time in Brooklyn. David took the risk of moving outside of his comfort zone. He told me he would sit at parties observing this crowd and wonder how these "poor and unattractive" people could seem so happy and full of life. I tried to withhold my distaste for that sentiment, because that question contained a profound realization for him: The answer was that they lived authentically, and he was inspired by a vitality that he had never felt. I remembered that dull look in his eyes when I first met him, the lifelessness behind his bravado. That had finally disappeared. David had begun to step beyond the illusions and narrow confines of his ego. He could actually just consider what *he* wanted.

I had him continually ask himself: What does my ego want?

What do I want? Eventually, David made several big decisions. He was *not* ready to get married or to buy a house in Westchester. He stayed on Wall Street, but he broke up with Nikki and actually moved to Brooklyn. He started spending his free time learning how to play the guitar instead of collecting numbers in bars. He read books and went to museums. We spent our time talking about all of his new discoveries, which were both banal and profound.

I worked with David for more than a year and watched his slow but gratifying transformation. And my own reaction to David had also evolved from a place of fear and knee-jerk disgust to a deep compassion for a very human struggle.

Men like David, who womanize, tend to be quickly categorized with pejorative labels like "pig" or "jerk," and it's easy to judge and hate them. And yet this womanizing behavior is motivated by the same core emotional needs of love, trust, and acceptance that drive us all in often very illogical and dysfunctional ways.

In this regard, we are all David.

I don't know if David ever found love, but I do know that he had begun the lifelong journey of learning to love himself. Ironically, we did little over the course of our sessions to actually *define* what love is. In fact, I think we did more to define what love is not. You have to start somewhere. But I do know, as he put it in our first session, that David was now doing a fine job preparing himself to become "capable of love."

This examination of love, however, was not over for me.

RAMI

I met Rami while working on my doctorate in Florida. At the time, I waited on tables a few nights a week at a Lebanese restaurant. Rami was a regular customer, and a friend of the owner, but to me he was just another unfocused face as I rushed by taking orders and delivering food.

The night we met, Rami sat with a raucous group at a big table in my section. Later, I would learn that they had sat there intentionally. I was very busy, and I didn't sense his eyes on me as I weaved in and out of tables, grabbing bites of food and sips of wine from regular customers. Rami and his friends were smoking hookahs and taking turns getting up to dance with the belly dancer. After dinner, I saw them heatedly engaged in a classic Middle Eastern melodrama: fighting over who gets the honor of paying the check. As I walked past the commotion, Rami grabbed my wrist and asked for my phone number. Outright. No small talk or flattery; he simply got right to the point with a tactic that seemed straight from a poorly skilled womanizer-wannabe's repertoire. And yet something about his tone was unexpectedly friendly, even earnest. And his eyes were so alive that the question actually sounded more natural than offensive.

I wish I could say it was a heart-stopping moment, but it wasn't. He'd just caught me off guard as my mind raced: Table eleven needs a refill; that chicken shwarma is probably up in the kitchen; table three needs their check. I'd never even spoken to this guy and he already wanted my phone number? Awkward.

However, a big table equals a big tip, and they hadn't paid yet, so I gave him my stock answer for forward customers I'd rather not embarrass in front of their friends: "Sure. Just call me here at the restaurant," I said, then shimmied away with a smile.

Rami returned the next morning while I helped set up tables for lunch. "Let me just take you out to breakfast." His easy charm suggested that I would be silly to resist an invitation so harmless.

Maybe it was Rami's beguiling smile, but I agreed.

"Good. I'll pick you up tomorrow morning at eleven," he said, before walking off to chat up some of the other waitresses, all of whom clearly enjoyed his attentions. I, on the other hand, felt like I had been smoothly conned into buying a product I didn't want. How did that happen? It wasn't like me to fold so easily, and moreover, Rami's type had never registered on my datable radar. He was at least ten years my senior—maybe more.

As I watched him talk to my coworkers, I took a moment to study this man who I thought was probably just a benign nuisance. Tall, with rugged Mediterranean features and intense black eyes, Rami had a strong jaw, olive skin, and dark, wavy hair with flecks of gray. He seemed exotic, sophisticated, and slightly subversive. I imagined that he drank expensive scotch and smoked cigars. I had to admit that he *was* sexy in a classic old movie star way, like Clark Gable or Omar Sharif.

The next morning over breakfast, Rami told me his life story. He told me how he had grown up in West Bank refugee camps in the Palestinian territory and now owned commercial real estate throughout the U.S. South. He'd emigrated to the States in his early twenties and was now retired at age forty. He spent most of his time traveling and had homes in Morocco and Spain. "I go several times a year," he explained. "Some of my friends also own homes and vacation there."

I'd never met anyone like Rami. My previous boyfriend was a Bohemian counterculture type who drove an old VW bus and walked around without shoes. He was sweet, wonderful, and loving. We'd been together for six years, until I left because he'd become more of a brother than a lover. I was more ambitious and had bigger plans, and I was ready to date a different type of man: someone who would challenge me, stimulate me. Rami brought a new excitement to my life, and I jumped into a fast and intense relationship with him.

Rami was able to offer something even more seductive to me than money or handsome looks; he could offer adventure. I think this was compelling for me because I came from a conservative background. My family still lives in the small, pretty Southern town where I grew up. As an adult, I can now see the beauty of that simple existence. But as a teenager, my parents' lifestyle seemed too narrow. I was restless with wanderlust. Maybe it was the World Book encyclopedia set my dad bought me as a child, with all those pictures of the Amazon and the Far East, because even as an adult, my attraction to the exotic never faded.

Rami and I came from different worlds, had different religions and cultural traditions. I loved the differences even though I didn't fully understand them. In fact, I probably fetishized the differences rather than realizing that some measure of similarity is fundamental to a relationship.

As I fell in love with Rami, some of my friends, seeing only visions of turbans and terrorists, worried about my burgeoning interest in Arabic culture. But I felt as if I had stepped through a magic portal onto the old silk trade route. He took me to dance to arabesque music, we smoked apple hookahs, drank spicy teas, and traveled the Middle East. Our romance literally flowered against the heady backdrop of voluptuous pillows and rich fabrics draped over low-slung couches made for lying in repose while eating figs and waiting to be made love to. Our courtship was a feast for the senses with the ever-present aromas of cumin, nutmeg, and allspice, and the rhythm of soft tribal drumbeats, and songs with throaty voices of longing and haunting airy flutes.

I was dazzled by this world and the way that it expanded me. My mother was concerned. She predicted that I would eventually realize that Rami and I weren't a match. We were "unequally yoked" she would say.

I wasn't concerned given that neither of us was religious—despite the notable exception of a canoe trip down a river in Florida one summer when an afternoon thunderstorm erupted and caught us in the middle of the waterway, cowering while lightning bolts crashed all around us. We began to paddle as fast as we could to get off the river, while I called out to Jesus and he to Allah. When we made it to the riverbank, I asked Rami, "Why do you call yourself a Muslim? You don't go to the mosque, you don't observe Ramadan—well you go to the dinners, but you also eat all day—and you went to a Catholic school growing up."

"I was born Muslim," he said.

"But you're not born religious," I said.

"Yes, but I was born into a religious culture," he replied.

I did notice that Rami practiced the most beautiful parts of Islam. He measured himself by his hospitality, generosity, and acceptance of others—particularly the poor. He spent a great deal of his time volunteering at a soup kitchen for the homeless, and if he felt inspired, he turned his own house into a soup kitchen. He once collected a crew of domestic and lawn workers from his property, cooked a full-on feast, and then served it to them in his dining room. They were bemused. I really appreciated how much he enjoyed giving to others, and whether this was religion or his personality, I chose to focus on this virtue rather than any differences between us.

So I went about my usual pattern of glamorizing love and dolling it up in a provocative dress, never wanting to look for any imperfections beneath the surface. I didn't want any unseemly information interrupting my reverie. Maybe there were differences, but they didn't seem to matter.

Until about four months into our courtship, when he invited me along on a trip to Morocco with his friends.

In a dimly lit and crowded Marrakech restaurant, the sound of live drums and clanging zills filled the air as the belly dancers shimmied seductively by. Rami had brought me to a place where he and his group of Arab-American businessmen friends—some of whom owned houses in the area—often came to party. We sat down to a feast of couscous and, to my surprise, an assortment of girls as young as thirteen and as old as seventeen.

I was immediately and deeply uncomfortable. Was I watching sexual tourism in action? I realized that each man would take one or several girls with him for the evening.

I studied these girls. They looked young and yet prematurely aged. One seemed like a scrappy street kid, hungry and hypervigilant, eyes darting. She bent over her food in a primal position, cupping the couscous with her hands while periodically peering over her shoulder. Next to her was a quiet girl, with good manners. But her erect posture and clenched hands failed to conceal her unease. Another girl, whose clothing was a poor attempt at Western fashion, was quite coquettish and would have been remarkably beautiful if not for overt signs of malnutrition.

Did my male companions not understand that they were exploiting young girls in a desperate economic situation? Did they not care about the physical and emotional collateral damage?

On a trip to the restroom, I started talking to the coquettish girl. I wanted to find out why she was with these men. The truth was unsettling. The girls weren't victims of human trafficking, sold via organized crime or even a local pimp. They'd been sent by their families, and they in fact did dream of marrying a French tourist or becoming the second wife of a Saudi businessman so that they could provide money for their entire family. In the meantime, they would settle for some food, a little money, or a pair of pants. She explained, in halting English, that with employment opportunities so limited, and no sexual harassment laws to protect women in the work environment, they were always vulnerable to being coerced to have sex with their male coworkers.

These girls had no options, no protection, and no voice. I sensed an overwhelming feeling of resignation and hopelessness in them, despite their masks of charm and ease. I understood that the culture was not my own, but I also believed that beneath the surface, mental gymnastics were likely needed to make their reality tolerable. I imagined that they had to shut down their authentic feelings and were robbed of basic relational needs like trust, safety, and love. It seemed to me that this wasn't simply the age-old exchange of sex for money, but that instead whatever exchange was taking place was at the expense of the young girls' sense of dignity and humanity.

I couldn't stand it any longer. I stood, glared at Rami, and said "I'm going to call the American embassy, and I'm going to go home." I was speaking loudly. His friends overheard, and they looked at me as if I were terminally naïve. And yet they spouted justification upon justification. "We are *helping* these girls and their families," said one. Another vilified the girls as complicit tricksters out to scam men into marriage. Rami desperately tried to reassure me that he had never participated in his friends' misadventures. It took much ministration from him to calm me. Yet in that moment, it finally became undeniable to me that Rami and I had very different perspectives on love and relationships.

When I'd met Rami, he lived alone. He spent most of his time with this group of friends, throwing parties and traveling together like a middle-aged fraternity. In truth, Rami and his friends were libertines who lived an epicurean lifestyle of luxury and hedonism, free of any constraints. This was what they believed in. Some of Rami's friends liked to provoke me into philosophical debates. The Great Love versus Libertine debates as I liked to refer to them. "What's the point of romantic love?" or "Why would I want to spend all of my time with a woman?" they would ask me as if they were trying to understand a completely ridiculous way of looking at the world. They really didn't trust in love; they saw it as an illusion at best and a constraint at worst. To these men, the only truth was physical pleasure. Women were part of life's riches, just like food or fine wine.

At first I wondered if their attitude toward love had everything to do with their cultural origins, where marriage was sometimes a business arrangement. I noticed that they didn't expect romance or even friendship in a partnership. But I also knew from their stories that they had all been friends since childhood, and while growing up they had participated in nonviolent protests against the loss of their homes, attempts at changing the world that had only landed them in prison on various occasions, so they left for America to make it in business. They had all abandoned their former life of high ideals, principle, justice, etc., and taken on a point of view that it's naïve to think you can change the world, so just enjoy life. And now they were living that dream—though I thought they seemed empty and depressed. I was really struck by that. So much freedom and money, yet they weren't full of vigor and joy like Rami and I were at the time, which left Rami caught in between these two philosophies.

I think our sheer ebullience about each other silently won that debate, and as a result, Rami's friends took an adversarial attitude toward me—as a way of venting disapproval that their most gregarious single friend would bring me along to everything—every dinner, every party, every trip. I was a real spoiler for these guys. They'd speak only Arabic, intentionally leaving me out of the conversation.

I decided to outsmart them. I went to Barnes & Noble and found a dictionary of Egyptian Arabic. I studied it in secret so that when Rami and his pals switched languages I would be able to pick up bits of the conversation. Sounds like a tall order, but I have a keen talent for memorizing. I carried that book everywhere and read it whenever possible—on subways, in line for coffee, while brushing my teeth, etc. I also practiced where and whenever I could, like with the Egyptian man who worked at the halal street cart on a corner near my apartment, and I'd try to give directions to cabbies from the Middle East.

One afternoon, while sitting in a coffee shop with Rami and friends, I spoke up. I don't remember my exact words, but I do remember their reaction: shock and surprise, followed by laughter. "She's speaking Arabic! *Egyptian* Arabic!"

I hadn't realized there were different dialects. Yet I earned their grudging respect, and they began to speak to me occasionally in Arabic. Rami decided to teach me his dialect, spending many hours with me lounging in bed in various states of undress, playing word games. I found the language to be very seductive, a series of guttural tones, coming from deep in the throat, emotional, somehow closer to the soul. The language didn't seem to allow for restraint, leaving me feeling both bolder and more exposed as I tried to express myself. The cadence was rough, raw, and inharmonious, with inflections that only added passion and intensity to any expression. It's a language that is particularly erotic in a man's deep, raspy voice. Then there was this one unique letter, a softer sound that stood out, one I so loved to hear from Rami's lips, a sort of breathy, elongated H—the kind of sound one would make when exasperated or overcome with pleasure. And when interpreted, even ordinary expressions were full of ornate poetry and spirituality. Lovers addressed each other with words like *RoHi,* with that breathy H, which meant, "my soul," or *Naseebi*, which meant "my destiny." But my two favorite words were *Habibi*, "my love," and *ya-la*, "let's go." I delighted in calling everyone *Habibi* for a couple of years.

I worried at times about the influence of Rami's friends, but much to their chagrin, Rami remained loyal to me and seemed to enjoy flaunting our togetherness in their presence.

And soon, one night as he thought I was sleeping, he tenderly stroked my hair and whispered, *"Ana b'Hybek"* ("I love you"). And I was falling in love with him. I looked him in the eyes and said "Let's love each other with abandon. Let's not guard off any parts of ourselves, let's feel this love as deeply as we can." These words were important to me. I believed that so much adult love came packaged in protective layers, and I wanted to take the risk to be completely open, to forgo that fearful need for safety and to fully experience our feelings.

When Rami and I became a couple, my coworkers at the restaurant acknowledged his charm, but they also murmured about his freewheeling lifestyle and, one night, his marital status. That made me wonder for a moment, but no one knew anything for certain. He had told me that he was divorced, and frankly I had no reason not to believe him. I was reassured that Rami was always available, and we regularly spent the night at his place, which looked like a typical very lived-in bachelor pad.

But Rami was also irrepressibly gregarious, charming, and an insatiable flirt. More and more I began to notice what my friends were talking about. One evening, we were at a formal dinner. I was all dressed up and felt beautiful. Then a stunning young woman Rami knew walked by. He got excited, jumped out of his seat, kissed her cheek, and said, "Can I send a bottle of wine to your table?" He made a big deal over her, then sat down. Twenty minutes later, another woman he knew walked past and he did the same thing. I felt a pang of jealousy.

Later, at his house, I gave in to an irresistible urge to confront him.

"You're flirting with other women."

"I'm just friendly. It means nothing."

"You seem to know a lot of women. How do you know all these women?"

He shrugged. What could he say? I kept going. "You know, the people at the restaurant always talk about you."

"They're just friends."

"I keep hearing things."

He took the bait. "What things?"

"Well . . . someone told me that you're married."

Rami shook his head. "Absolutely not. I'm divorced. I told you."

I stared him in the eyes.

"It's an . . . Islamic divorce," he said.

A what? "What does *that* mean?"

"It's Islamic . . . cultural . . . not . . . legal. But it's the same thing," he added quickly.

"So, you're *not* divorced!"

Rami wore a baleful look. "I've wanted to tell you so often, but the time just didn't seem right. Here's the story. It was a strategic marriage. Not arranged, but practical for both parties. You have to understand, in my culture, marriage isn't always about love. We've been separated for six years and she lives in another state."

All the air went out of me. I couldn't believe he had waited until I fell in love with him to tell me the truth. Was anything Rami had told me true? I wanted him to take it all back, to say something, anything, to make everything okay.

"Why didn't you ever tell me?"

"I wanted to, but I was afraid you wouldn't understand."

"I wouldn't have dreamed of getting involved with a married man."

"See? I wanted to give us a chance first."

"I think you just blew that chance."

Rami scrambled to explain, saying that he and his wife had mutually agreed to separate but not divorce, for financial reasons. As a result, he'd hook up with random women, but he never went out with anyone for too long because he didn't want to find a serious relationship and then have a woman request that he get divorced. If he could see that a woman was getting emotionally involved with him, he would break up with her. "But you are different," he said. "I feel like I've fallen in love for the first time."

I had to get away. I went home and the next day I broke it off. Very soon I'd head to New York alone to start my postgraduate internship.

I wanted to live in Manhattan and couldn't afford it on my own. I needed a roommate. I was introduced to young woman named Sophie who was also moving to New York alone at the same time. We flew there together to look for a place to live. A broker showed us around, but we couldn't find anything that worked. We returned home frustrated and, in my case, a little nervous because my internship would start soon.

I went on Craigslist and found one room in a five bedroom railroad apartment for $800 a month. There were no pictures, but I was desperate enough to rent it sight unseen. I called Sophie and said, "Let's just get this room and share it." I mailed the subletter money, and he said I could move in.

I showed up by myself and saw a flat brick building on 30th Street and Fifth Avenue. Each floor had one apartment. I walked up to the fifth floor, knocked on the door, and a man opened it. He wore an ill-fitting suit, had big bushy hair, and I thought he looked kind of creepy. In accented English he introduced himself as Nestor. "Hi. You live here," he said, and walked me through the narrow living room, past a dirty, old couch and a tiny TV, and down a cramped dark hallway to my "room." It was empty. No closet. "Sometimes I also stay here . . . on the couch," he added, hoping that it wouldn't be a problem for me. Nestor showed me three outfits that he kept in a little utility closet. He also pointed out the kitchenette and a door that led to a fire escape.

Sophie showed up a week later. "What the hell is this place?" she shrieked.

Including myself and Sophie, ten people—both male and female—and several mice lived in the apartment, with Nestor occasionally on the couch. The apartment was clearly a large flat, and Nestor had put up cheap walls to make rooms, with no air-conditioning. The place was dirty and crowded. We had one bathroom with a phone booth–sized shower stall. You couldn't even change your clothes inside, it was so small.

With no closet in our room, Sophie and I put up bars around the perimeter, hung our clothes, and slept on the floor underneath them, on pillows. We couldn't afford a bed; any extra money went for clothes and good times. Our shoes and accessories were spread everywhere. It was like sleeping on the floor of a giant walk-in closet. We did have a big window, though, and we would lie in front of it at night talking, in the glow of the city lights—no curtains, of course—with our view of the Empire State Building. Sometimes a hot Brazilian guy who also lived there came in to lie around with us, laughing and talking about everything. We were, as I quickly discovered, just random young men and women who'd come to New York from around the world, for our educations and jobs, hoping to make it.

Sometimes friends visiting from Florida would ask how I could live that way, in the heart of Manhattan, on $12,000 a year—the stipend I got for my internship. I just said that the city was my living room. I fancied myself a modern Holly Golightly. I was actually quite happy.

Six months later Rami called. He wanted to get back together. He reiterated that he and his wife lived in different states, with no likelihood of reconciliation. They were bound only by paperwork. They both had shares in his business and agreed that to change that would be financially unwise. Everything about the "unofficial divorce" was amicable and agreed on by her.

Still, Rami had lied to me. However, I continued to love him, and I wanted to take risks for this thing called love that I had so professed to believe in during all of those wild debates with his friends.

We reconciled and commenced a long-distance relationship, once again blissfully in love. He tried to make up for his lie by pampering me. For example, one evening I came home and found Rami at my apartment, charming all of my girlfriends. He'd flown in to surprise me. He'd brought groceries to stock our fridge. "This is for all of you," he said. Then he cooked us an over-the-top dinner. He made my roommates laugh. After dinner he disappeared into the bathroom, where I caught him on his hands and knees cleaning the bathtub. Later I discovered that he'd hand-washed my delicates! And had folded my laundry. I'm not kidding. He behaved like this all the time. I will never find this again, I thought.

Rami easily won over my girlfriends because he wasn't acting. Rami could be a loving, protective, and caring man. On another evening my girlfriends were all grousing about how they'd gained weight, or saying they didn't like their hair, or imagining what kind of plastic surgery they wished they could get. Rami sat there, absorbing the chatter. Then he said, "Well, I don't care what Brandy looks like. I just love her. If she gained a hundred pounds or if she lost an arm, I would still go to the moon for her."

I promised Rami that I would come back to Florida in one year. Meanwhile, we moved forward—albeit erratically. Our relationship was like theater—we often lived in a state of high drama or being high *on* drama—and even we were entertained by it. I would say, "Remember that time I jumped out of the car in Morocco, in the middle of nowhere, and you left me? Or the time when you walked out on me at a restaurant because you thought I smiled at another man?" And then we'd both laugh and be filled with warmth and love, though I was often anxious about what Rami might be doing with his good old libertine friends when we were apart. Still, Rami and I tried to see each other every two weekends. He'd fly north or I'd fly south. But in between, I got lost in my head and often couldn't quit obsessing. My best girlfriend, weary of all of my Rami stories, just shook her head and said, "One of you two is gonna have a stroke."

I didn't see it clearly at the time, but my ruminations always led back to the soul-crushing revelation of him not telling me the truth about his marital arrangement. That betrayal of trust was what first sent our relationship off the tracks—and I became extra wary. I wasn't in any hurry to get married, so I wanted to just live with it, but the seed had been planted. That moment probably set the tone for everything that followed.

I'd wonder if we were right for each other. I'd wonder if he saw other women. I'd analyze the good times and the bad, and agonize about which pointed toward the truth. I'd scribble in my diaries. I'd explain—and then explain away—the feeling in the pit of my stomach every time my emotions veered crazily. After I started my own practice, especially in the early going, I'd sometimes lose focus for a second while listening to my patients' problems, because hearing truths about men, from men, made me think of Rami and things that would upset any woman.

Even outside the office, my mind was always busy. I started to make lists. Good qualities versus bad qualities. I searched for a narrative, a story to tell myself about the relationship, so that my emotional reactions would be at least consistent. One day I'd be convinced that Rami was a womanizer and the next that he was simply a friendly guy. Or that he was a pathological liar, or just trying to impress me, keep me around, or protect me. Or that his lying wasn't so bad, but actually kind of flattering and endearing.

And I could as easily turn my list-making on myself: Am I just focusing on the negative and ignoring the positive? Am I creating my own headache? He is wonderful. I am crazy. Time to shut my diary. Good night.

I wanted to find one simple question I could ask myself that would end my internal battle. Call it the golden question that would determine if I should stay or go. I read a relationship column that asked, "Does he add to your life force or take it away?" This resonated. My sparkle, my spirit had been regularly inflated then deflated.

My mom asked, "Do you enjoy his company? If you're going to spend all your days with one person, what matters is that you truly enjoy his company."

A friend asked, "Is he going to take care of you financially?"

I asked myself, "Is this love or fantasy? Is this about love or my ego? Why am I really with him?"

ALEX

"I met the Russian at a quiet basement lounge in Chelsea. We sat in the corner near the fireplace, deep in conversation about a book I'd read on freedom of speech in the Ukraine. He said he was a diplomat, but I thought he might be a clandestine agent as well."

This was my first meeting with Kasha. She was the girlfriend of Alex, my patient of two months. She was originally from Brazil, and had high cheekbones and almond-shaped eyes that she enhanced with dark eyeliner extending past the corners, adding to her exoticism. Kasha was rhapsodizing about a recent encounter in florid detail.

"His dark and intense eyes pulled me in," she continued, with a mild accent, but without pause or reservation. "It was as if he was trying to—I don't know—find me behind my words as I questioned him. I couldn't believe we were actually sitting together, and I wondered if he could tell that I was trembling, longing for him.

"He must have, because suddenly he slowly began to run his finger along the outline of my lips, and stopped my inquiries by gently inserting his finger into my mouth.

"We left the bar and went to his hotel room at the Soho Grande. I was . . . I wanted to be . . . ravaged. Immediately. Yet, he made me wait. His voice was soft, slow, and firm, as he told me to sit on the bed and unbutton my blouse. I did, while he watched from across the room, nodding with approval as my breasts were bared. I kept undressing and he called my every curve magnificent. Finally, he came closer, and as I lifted my skirt to expose my thighs, he pulled my panties to my knees. He put his lips at my ear and whispered, "Good girl." I heard his belt unbuckle. I felt my panties pulled all the way down, and I kicked them away. With my blouse still hanging from my shoulders, he gripped the back of my hair, looked me in the eyes, and began to penetrate me, hard and slow.

"Can you see now why I don't want to fuck my boyfriend?" Kasha asked, softly.

Uh, yes. I could.

Kasha had hypnotized me with her bodice-ripping tale. Not that I could luxuriate in the afterglow with her. Instead, I had to shake off the hot flush and regain my therapeutic distance. I was also baffled by this seductive recounting of events for a very different reason. Kasha was nothing like the woman Alex had prepped me to meet. According to him, she was an asexual granny pants. After dating for three years, Alex had come to me concerned that Kasha had grown averse to sex. He wanted to resurrect her fading libido and keep them from slipping into one of those complacent, desexualized relationships we all read about in women's magazines.

After a few sessions on our own, Alex couldn't wait to suggest a meeting with Kasha. He had no gut-whispering idea that he was being cheated on. However, I could see a clear, deep chasm between reality and his perception. I felt credulous for buying into Alex's tale of their relationship, and chagrined at Kasha as well, on his behalf, as if I, too, had been betrayed.

Kasha was a blunt reminder that I can never allow myself to be pulled completely into a patient's narrative as if it represents the truth.

I try not to judge, but even before I met Kasha, I had worried that poor Alex didn't have a sexy bone in his body. Alex was a research scientist at a pharmaceutical company. He seemed a strange, elfish creature in his practical khaki trousers, button-down shirts, and thin-rimmed glasses. I imagined that his sense of security relied on concrete terms, measurements, numbers, lists, organization.

When he'd come in to talk about Kasha, Alex was purposeful and tense, and tried in vain not to seem anxious. He constantly adjusted his glasses and ran his fingers down a pant leg crease. His foot shook, and he crossed his leg over his knee to hold it still. At the same time he waited expectantly with a notepad and pen, like an eager student.

I have always instinctively wanted to root for or defend patients like Alex. He was an overly intellectual, pedantic guy, confident in his arcane knowledge, a classic nerd. But rather than aloof and remote, he came across as endearing and eager to please. He might know a lot about many things, but he was still innocent and earnest about relationships.

Alex opened by telling me that he'd called me because he'd done research and knew that I had specialized in women with low sexual desire. True, I said, and told him that it was women's most ubiquitous sexual complaint and, ironically, an issue for which they didn't often seek treatment. While women are more inclined than men to seek psychotherapy for depression or anxiety, grief or marital conflicts, when it comes to sexual desire they often assume that the decline is normal.

After meeting Kasha, I couldn't imagine that she and Alex knew each other, much less belonged together; they were so different. But they'd been together for three years. Kasha liked to write about politics and wanted more recognition. She said she'd been attracted to Alex's stability and respected his intellect. His wealth of knowledge stimulated and inspired her. She was ambitious; he was grounded. He preferred structure and routine. She was more restless.

Alex and Kasha shared a one-bedroom apartment in an Upper West Side brownstone. Previously she'd lived in Queens. That, she said, had been an uncertain time, full of both self-doubt and hope. With Alex, Kasha saw herself as part of a quintessential young intellectual couple officially integrated into New York culture. They had interesting friends, loved literature, poetry, and politics, and every morning they read the *New York Times* together over coffee and bagels.

I wondered how much of Kasha's attraction to Alex was based on her needs at the time they'd met. While this is to some extent true of all couples, in Kasha's case I believed that while her move to New York reflected her penchant for adventure and novelty, she also immediately needed to feel safe and secure in other ways in order to explore that penchant. Alex gave her that, and having since adjusted, she'd become bored with him and now needed more stimulation. Alex was convenient for a while, but a connection can't be built on such temporary motivations unless the relationship grows and more commonality is discovered.

When Alex suggested that I meet Kasha, he wanted a joint session. I asked to see her alone first, as I often do. That unencumbered time seemed the best way to get her side of the story. And I had. In lurid detail. But now, due to the ethics of doctor-patient confidentiality, I had to hold the heaviness of her secret life and keep her truth carefully compartmentalized—just as she did. Looking Alex in the eyes, I felt complicit in his betrayal.

I met with Kasha again and wanted to assess her commitment to the relationship before broaching the possibility of her revealing her affair to Alex.

"I want to stay with him, yes," she said. "But to be honest, I'm not *that* attracted to him. I want to make it work because I know I've found a good man. I can trust him and he treats me well. But sometimes the relationship feels more like he's a brother or a good friend. But I suppose this happens in all relationships," she said with a confident and stony resignation, a real cynicism that revealed itself from behind her lively effrontery. It's interesting, I thought, to watch people brace themselves for what they believe to be some sad reality of life, harnessing their souls into a grim acceptance.

"Yeah, but what if this is it?" I prodded. I wanted to align with her pessimism and agitate her more. "What if less desire is just a natural part of relationships?"

"God, how boring," Kasha responded, tossing her hair and rolling her eyes. "Yes, I feel content and safe, but there is no fire. I need fire. I can't live like this forever!"

This was the great dilemma of monogamy. Kasha didn't want to make a choice between security and passion. This existential quandary presents the ultimate trade-off, the thought of a life without either eliciting paralyzing fear. Many people choose to cut off passion, or maybe, in an attempt to honor their own life force, they look for it somewhere outside of their primary relationship. However, I wasn't so sure this was a real dilemma. Maybe it was a false choice.

That very quandary was at the heart of the research that had resulted, a few years prior, in my dissertation on the topic of women's low libido. In my review of the relevant research, I discovered that withering sexual desire was considered an epidemic among women and, more surprising to me, one of the few sexual issues that didn't have any effective treatment. This wasn't an issue I'd confronted personally at the time; in fact, I could barely identify with what I was studying. I was alive with the euphoria of a brand-new romance with Rami. The inevitable demise of sexual desire that I had heard people speak of represented to me a perdition of the soul. I couldn't accept that passionate relationships are destined to burn out and that if I wanted a long-term relationship I would have to trade passion for safety. But why no effective treatment? Was it all just a lost cause or, worse, natural? This really made me curious. Perhaps I could learn something from my own level of desire.

I decided to start with the attitude that there *was* something I can do to maintain desire in my own relationship, that I wouldn't be inert, another hapless victim of the safety-versus-fire dichotomy, that I would take charge of this, make it my responsibility to maintain the flow.

On a trip to Morocco with Rami, I took a pile of Xeroxed journal articles and book chapters on women's sex drive—largely written by men, I noted—and read through them as Rami and I drove from Fez to Marrakech.

We were at the height of our love. It felt gloriously irrational. I loved him with fervor and awe. I didn't want it to end. I remember sitting next to him in the car, just staring at the shape of his lips and the small gap between his front two teeth, lost in his beauty as he talked to me. I couldn't stop touching him—his olive skin, his thick dark hair. I was literally petting him, pressing my hands into his flesh as though I wanted to feel something beyond it, and still I wasn't close enough. I wanted to get inside of his mind, explore and occupy each part of it. I wanted to live in all of his memories, to steal them and insert myself into them. I wanted to go back in time to when he was a little boy and live in his village, starve with him, and sleep next to him in the one-room refugee camp shelter that was his home.

At the time, we had only been dating for five months and I was in my last year of graduate school. Although I was usually very focused in class, I'd lately had a hard time concentrating because I couldn't stop daydreaming about Rami. I'd picture the way he'd made love to me the night before, or what I anticipated for later that day. When sex is that good, it can distract you from anything.

The frequency of my fantasies about Rami only increased my

desire, and I realized that this was something I could control. Not to stop it, but to stay in a highly stimulated state. Of course, these sexual thoughts came naturally at the time to someone in the throes of new love, but I wondered if I could also choose them anytime, at will. Could I continue to make myself see the world sexually? When I used to tell Rami, "You are so beautiful," he would say, "No, it's your eyes that see me as beautiful." Maybe he had a point. Perception could be manipulated. Could I be the source of sexual inspiration and not simply respond when Rami inspired it? Men do it all the time, I thought, why don't women?

I decided to track my ability to do this, making my relationship into sort of a laboratory—and it worked.

But I also noticed obstacles to my strategy: Emotional junk and other, usually negative thoughts and images could block my ability to hold on to this sexualized view of the relationship.

I remembered reading an article on that trip about a phenomenon researchers had labeled the "sexual intimacy paradox." They had discovered that marital therapy strategies designed to increase emotional intimacy were correlated with a decline in sexual desire. Further, they cited other studies that reported that couples therapy techniques designed to improve communication skills and overall relationship quality were at times associated with an increase in sexual problems. What? They found that couples with the most egalitarian, communicative, and comfortable relationships had the least amount of passion. But factors responsible for *increasing* libido were distance, novelty, danger, and power differences.

That didn't sound like good news at all for long-term relationships.

I never take any one study or even a series of studies too seriously, because when you read so many articles they all end up reporting opposing results and nullifying one another. But I couldn't help wonder how this concept applied to Kasha and Alex. They had that comfortable, egalitarian type of relationship that looks like it should work; however Kasha wanted something more. Had the new sense of adventure drawn her into her affair? I wanted to find out what she was really looking for. What were all the possible ingredients of this tenuous potion we call sexual desire?

"Tell me about sex with Alex," I asked Kasha

"We had chemistry in the beginning, but now it's faded, very, very dim," she continued. Kasha made a small space between her thumb and forefinger to illustrate her point. She described Alex as "tender and gentle," and their lovemaking as "mostly missionary," but said that for a long time she didn't mind because she felt loved. "He'd kiss me deeply, look into my eyes, hold me. Alex's warmth made me feel very secure and that was very satisfying."

Kasha frowned.

"But?"

"But over time it just seemed that he wanted it more than I did. I'd have been happy to do it once a week, but he wanted sex every night. I'd be tired from working all day and want to go to bed early, but he'd want sex."

"How did that make you feel?"

"Irritated, to be honest. I'd just do it to get it over with. No big deal at first, but eventually I started resisting. And he would *still* try, which turned me off even more. Now I've just lost interest completely."

"So, by saying yes when you didn't want to have sex, a loving act was turned into a duty or obligation."

"I believe you have to keep a man happy, so he doesn't cheat," she snapped.

"Do you really think it makes Alex happy when you comply with sex you don't want?"

"Of course. He has no idea. I have my fantasies. I put on a performance. I groan a little, squirm, and fake an orgasm if necessary. No harm done."

Perfectly logical according to Kasha, but I recognized this as the first stage in a typical pattern that plunges couples into sexual desolation. When sex becomes "duty sex," then it's a chore, a task, an item on the to-do list. At best you're detached; at worst you're resentful. Where's the natural enjoyment?

Kasha's tone with me was a bit condescending. She spoke with a confidence that suggested she was letting me in on some ancient Brazilian wisdom about men. What Kasha didn't realize was that men are often painfully aware when women are not authentically engaged. In fact, Alex had described sex with Kasha during the past year as "soulless." Her kisses, he said, were perfunctory and impatient, her touch rigid and mechanical, her eyes empty, and her appearance at home dowdy—but sexy when she dressed for work. Despite Kasha's "performance," an emotional presence had evaporated. Alex reacted by trying harder to please Kasha. However, the more he strived, the less interested she became, and the more rejected he felt. He was desperate for any sign of warmth, and she experienced him as needy. Sensing her disconnected compliance, he began to rush through their encounters, thinking he was burdening her, and thus satisfying her even less.

"It's like having sex with a mannequin," Alex had told me. "She looks perfect and goes through the motions, but she's not actually alive."

Alex was angry about his lost connection with Kasha, but he never let her see his inner struggle. That would just make things worse, he thought. But finally, when his insecurity had grown intolerable, Alex came to me.

"So, no harm done to Alex, right?" I said, repeating Kasha's words back to her. I wished I could tell her that Alex was on to her artifice. Instead I turned it back on her. "What about the harm this charade does to you?"

Kasha smiled and coyly averted her eyes, but she didn't have an answer. It struck me then that no matter how she presented herself to Alex, no matter how expertly she went through the motions in bed, no matter how natural her beauty, Kasha lacked authentic sexual confidence. She simply acted the part.

"Don't *you* get bored pretending to be into it with Alex?" I said.

"I don't get bored with the Russian," she shot back.

I didn't ask what she liked most about being with the Russian. Hell, *I* thought the Russian sounded sexy.

"Do you feel like you are sexier with Alex or the Russian?"

"The Russian. Obviously."

"Why is that? I wonder. Why does that change for you based on who you're with?"

Kasha couldn't say—and the answer is not as obvious as you might think. In fact, her hot tryst with the Russian actually underscored my assessment that Kasha wasn't assertive. "When you described your encounter with the Russian, do you realize that your role was submissive? And with Alex it sounds passive. Where is *your* power in these interactions?"

In essence, I was really asking, "Where are you? And what do you want?"

"I have power!" Kasha insisted, vexed. "The power of having the Russian desire me, the power of keeping Alex's attention."

"You're describing validation not power," I said. "How about knowing what *you* want? What *you* need? What are *your* desires? *Your* turn-ons?"

Kasha retreated pensively. I sat quietly as she mulled over an answer. I hoped she'd open up, not shut down defensively.

"I don't know," she finally said.

This was exactly what I wanted her to realize. *She didn't know.* Yes, she was skilled in the art of seduction. She knew what *men* wanted, to a certain extent, but she had no idea what she wanted. Well, actually, she wanted to be wanted—and not much else—without having to do much. This is more of an *emotional* need, and the hallmark of a woman who would fall in to the trap of chronic low desire. Sex to validate one's ego alone is gratifying—but only temporarily. It doesn't sustain. I wanted to help Kasha to consider what *besides and beyond* validation might motivate her sexually. But first she had to realize that she *didn't know.*

"Knowing what you want is empowering, Kasha," I said, as we ended the session. "Knowing you don't know is a good beginning. We should start there next time."

Kasha seemed annoyed or perplexed, or both. And frustrated. She had no idea what this abstract concept of sexual motivation meant. But I knew she would reflect on our conversation. She was very analytical. However, I worried that she would be blinded by the instant excitement and sex appeal of the Russian.

I didn't want to beat up the girl for enjoying her own beauty and sexual prowess—trust me, I am all about celebrating both of these aspects of femininity. And it's true that women want sex more often when they feel sexy and desirable. But Kasha's affair was pandering to her narcissism, and her emphasis on admiration was blocking her ability to find other sources of sexual motivation. Kasha knew what *men* wanted, so she enhanced that look and enjoyed the attention. But it was still the fake sexiness of women who buy into generalized men's scripts. In a way it was like false advertising: She looks sexy, acts seductive, then once she lands the guy, she puts back on her retainer and glasses and hopes he doesn't bother her while she watches *Law & Order* reruns. Why? Because performing is exhausting, and eventually you want to relax and be yourself.

Alex was on to Kasha and so was I. He knew something was missing and he blamed himself. But he was only half of the equation. Even with the Russian, Kasha wasn't her true self. We all have the innate intelligence to know when something is inauthentic. Babies know when their mothers don't express love. My patients can tell when I don't care. Men aren't always turned on in strip clubs. (That's right. Men know it's just a show and would be far more turned on if the lap dancer *really* wanted them.)

I keep asking my patients a simple question that they often find difficult to answer: "What do you really want?"

Most don't know the answer, which means we have to spend serious time improving self-connection. But ultimately, I want to move my patients toward real expressions of love and lust: not a show, not a performance, no chimeras. It's amazing how many people *act* sexual or sexually and yet suppress or aren't familiar with their natural impulses. Kasha had no sense of her own natural eroticism because she was too wrapped up in the ego imperative of being desired. Sex can and does satisfy emotional needs. But sex isn't *just* emotional. It's physical as well: I wanted to help her find her lust, because lust is an important life force.

Kasha had no sense of her right to receive physical pleasure and to ask for it. This is a lesson that women can learn from men, who are socialized to have a sense of entitlement. Contrary to conventional wisdom, the men I've talked to are glad when women deviate from their sexual scripts, when they are not simply passive and receptive. They like a woman who knows what she wants and asks for it. They want to know that their partners have a strong sense of their own sexuality and enjoy experiencing it. All women need is to know who they are, and what they want, and not rely on men to do all the work and be responsible for their satisfaction.

Although I'd met with Kasha twice, she wasn't an official patient. Alex was, and I feared he was up against an almost impossible situation. Sex with Kasha had become routine, then almost nonexistent. Whose fault was it? I remembered what my mother used to say when I complained to her that I was bored: "Honey, if you're bored, that means you're boring."

In order to not be bored you need to take responsibility for your own enjoyment. The same applies to sex. They both had to work at it. But while Alex was confused about what to do, Kasha expected all of the excitement to come from the men she slept with. And in this case, poor Alex didn't have a chance against the Russian.

"I don't think Kasha loves me anymore," Alex said one day. Something had changed from the early sessions where he had felt safe enough with their relationship to suggest I meet with her. Now he was on a precipice, staring into a chasm of defeat, terrified of losing Kasha. My heart broke for him. "We're still best friends and we're affectionate, but there is no passion. She used to wear lingerie to bed and now it's T-shirt and boxers. She does nothing to show interest, she does nothing to seduce me anymore. She . . ."

I cut him off. "What do you do to seduce her?" I told him what my mother had said about boredom.

"Well . . . I try to give her an orgasm. I ask what I can do for her, but she doesn't respond. Really, it's the same routine every time. I kiss her, touch her breasts, rub her clit until she has an orgasm, then we have sex."

Alex confessed that he'd bought multiple self-help books on how to please a woman sexually but couldn't understand why the more he tried the techniques, the less Kasha was interested. I cringed silently at his hapless approach. No doubt most women, at one time or another, have endured the slow torture of monotonous sex.

"I can hear that you really want to please her."

"Yeah, desperately."

"And you believe that pleasing her means giving her an *orgasm*?" I hoped he had caught my mild sarcasm.

"She should be happy that I take care of her. Right?"

"Good sex is about more than orgasms."

Alex's eyes held a glimmer of understanding, but he couldn't put it all together. "It's like you have this goal-oriented approach," I continued. "I want you to throw away your encyclopedia's worth of female anatomical knowledge and sexual technique. Good sex is not an algorithm!"

Alex laughed self-consciously.

"It's the process! The dance around sex, the ceremony, the dynamic between the two of you that makes sex exciting."

I took a slim volume of poetry from my shelf. "I have a *new* instruction manual for you," I said, handing him the book. "Since you like poetry, take this. Pablo Neruda, *Captain's Verses*."

It was one of the hottest books I'd ever read. I didn't tell Alex that, because I hoped he'd discover it for himself. And perhaps he could absorb Neruda's example.

A Chilean poet and political activist, Neruda loved with authority, wore his vulnerability on his chest like a proudly decorated soldier, and spoke of his sexual desire in an unabashedly carnivorous manner. Neruda fled Chile when the Communists were being killed, and he wrote these poems while living in exile on the island of Capri. They were inspired by his wife, Matilde. That's right: animalistic and unrelenting desire, not for a mistress or a stranger, but for his wife. I thought the guy had something figured out.

Alex took the book, glanced at the cover, and stashed it in his bag.

"Let's look at your process as it stands now," I said. "I'm wondering if your attempts to please Kasha come off not as masterful but as servile and ingratiating."

I saw this all the time with my male clients: They learn some skills, but they don't have the chutzpah—self-possession and courage—to pull them off.

"Yeah," Alex said after a moment. "Probably not the sexiest qualities."

"How do you seduce her outside the bedroom?"

"I guess I didn't think I needed to make a conscious effort to seduce her. That sounds to me like trying too hard."

"Trying too hard?"

"If she loves me, it should just flow."

"That doesn't really work, Alex. You put effort into providing stability, friendship, and love. She is your best friend, but you're missing something. You must be a sexual object to her."

"A what?"

"That's right, Alex. *You* are a sex object!" I declared.

I know some may recoil at the phrase, but unless it's used as a single definition to subjugate you personally or politically, in the bedroom it's necessary. I wanted Alex to sexualize himself a bit. I still believed that Alex could be a *complete erotic lover* just as he was, if he was willing to take responsibility.

"Kasha is more than just your friend," I said. "She is your lover."

"And I want her to love me as I am," he said.

"That's not what I'm talking about," I said. "She is your *lover*."

I thought about Freud's concept of the incest taboo. Lovers become so enmeshed, so merged into their couplehood, that they start to see each other as family objects rather than sexual objects. They wind up desexualizing each other.

I wanted to give Alex a new frame of reference. I wanted him to go in the opposite direction and resexualize the relationship. This is what Neruda had done so well; he sexualized the hell out of his wife. He physically objectified her and loved her fiercely at the same time. It seemed Neruda had figured out how to have security—and passion—in a marriage.

Maybe Alex would respond to some visualization exercises, a way to turn some of his neurotic desperation into a positive. I have learned with patients that I can't impose my ideas of sexual fantasies on them; I have to let them start right where they are.

"Let's look at how we can work with what you feel right now. You're afraid of losing her. How does that feel in your body?"

"My stomach is tight."

"Can you imagine channeling that feeling of anxiety into passion, an intense hunger for Kasha?"

Alex shrugged, uncertain. I told him to close his eyes and asked what kind of feeling or fantasy came up.

"Sad. I wish I could keep her."

"Okay. Try to sexualize it. Use a little fantasy."

"I would . . . like to keep her in my apartment so she . . . doesn't run away. So she's only mine."

"Perfect. How will you make sure she doesn't get away?

"I can tie her up."

"Good, keep going."

"I'll tie her up and make her promise that she's mine. I'll fuck her as many times as I want."

"You will have her please you."

"Yes, I will feast on her body. I will bite her and mark her up."

I asked Alex how the exercise made him feel. "It made me horny," he said. Good. I wanted Alex to keep thinking that way, to convert all his fears into an empowered fantasy. We spent a few minutes doing this exercise during each of the next couple sessions, and I asked Alex to try it on his own. Finally, I suggested a homework assignment.

Alex was always the eager student and his malleability gave me room to teach him. Yet I worried I might set him up for failure. I was taking a chance here with my timing because Kasha might not be ready for Alex, given that she was so intoxicated by the Russian. But because I knew she still wanted her relationship with Alex to work, I thought it was worth the risk.

I told Alex that when he and Kasha got into bed that night he should tap the sexual energy and desire of his possession fantasy. "For example, take both of her hands behind her back and use your strength to restrain her and roll her on her side. I want you to talk softly into her ear and tell her that your love for her is so intense that you want to hold her captive and possess her. That she is so beautiful, you want her body only for you. Rub your body up against her. Grab a handful of her hair at the back of her head and kiss her passionately. Then stop. Don't initiate sex. Build her desire for you."

I had never suggested anything quite so detailed to a patient, but I thought Alex needed all the help he could get. I hoped to capitalize on his eagerness and viewed it as an opportunity to move beyond *talking* about sex with Alex and toward creating a *live experience* that would upset the couple's sexual homeostasis.

Of course, the bigger question was: Is it possible to teach a guy to be sexy? Most of sex therapy is oriented toward specific techniques that work on a physically identifiable dysfunction, like maintaining an erection or improving ejaculatory control. But I wasn't operating in the realm of the physical or the easily quantifiable; I wanted to help Alex create a new *attitude.* This was purely subjective; could he come to embody sex appeal?

I left my office, joyfully imagining that Alex would go home and really rouse Kasha out of her complacency. I felt imperious. I thought this intervention could be a real success.

When Alex came in the next week, I asked how his homework had gone.

"I didn't do it," he said.

My first instinct was to judge myself. Had I pushed my agenda before he was ready? Perhaps I had only increased his anxieties or set him up for rejection, although if this were true, I didn't perceive it as negative. Growth involves exposure to anxiety. I have noticed that in many of my cases, a "failed" homework assignment turns out to be successful for a different reason. Asking a client to act to his full potential will sometimes illuminate the real obstacle that needs to be addressed, by literally extracting it from the unconscious.

"I came up with a bunch of fantasies," he said. "Unfortunately, Kasha's been working on some story and wasn't home much. And when she got in, she was tired and went right to sleep. So there hasn't been a good time to do what you suggested."

"But at least you were creating fantasies. How did that part go for you?"

"I was nervous, but okay. It gives me another way to think about sex with Kasha."

"Any specific theme in the content of these fantasies?" Given the power aspects of his fantasy, I wanted to make sure he wasn't planning to act out anything violent or harmful.

"I just tried to figure out what I wanted. Mostly, I realized how long I'd been thinking *only* about what Kasha wants. So I've been imagining her pleasing me."

"How did that make you feel?"

"More confident in some ways.

"But . . . ?"

"Also uncomfortable that I was no longer thinking about pleasing her, too." Alex moved around on the couch trying to get comfortable. "I think of these fantasies . . . and then when I see Kasha lying in bed, even though I'm not going to do anything then, I freeze. I'm anxious that what I do will be so different from our routine. What's she going to think? I don't want her to think I'm just acting."

"That makes sense, Alex. But the problem is, you were acting *before*. Now you're actually trying to be authentic."

"That feels strange."

"That part where you felt confident," I said, as we wrapped up, "I need you to replay that in your mind, over and over."

How could I get Alex past his hang-up of worrying about what Kasha wanted or, worse, what she would think of him? He always put her first, and I wanted him to think of himself instead. Sure, she might wonder what's going on; she might not respond immediately, or ever. But if Alex couldn't overcome his fears and follow through, he'd have no chance of making changes, and the relationship would likely die.

I was surprised at how many of my male clients were anxious to the point of dysfunction over their desire to satisfy a woman. On one hand I took heart that men could sincerely value a woman's pleasure so much that they'd forget or postpone their own. But that could also turn pathetic if it was really all about an obsessive need to please and perform. What a situation: Men worried about pleasing women, while women were conflicted about their right to receive pleasure. An orgy of anxiety.

A girlfriend had recently told me that she'd started dating an attorney. He was very powerful at work, she said, but a "total wimp" with her. "He was so stiff and vanilla in bed that I took charge. I asked him to spank me. He couldn't do it. He froze. What the hell is going on with guys?"

Alex had an overdeveloped need to please, and I had to find a way to help him build a reservoir of self-confidence that could douse the fires of his anxiety and help Kasha rekindle her libido. Alex certainly played a role in Kasha's low libido. His nightly pursuit of sex was coming from a place of feeling anxious about their connection and needing reassurance. Her sexual compliance symbolically represented that she still wanted him, but she was turned off by his neediness.

Sometimes thinking about the whole dynamic exhausted me. Who needs all these complications around the simple act of inserting the penis into the vagina? Why do we have to analyze it? Sex is sex. It's simple.

Only it isn't.

We are humans. We attach meaning to sex, fulfill psychological needs with sex, and use sex as a tool to get what we want. That's what makes the topic interesting. If sex were just sex, it would be boring. When researching women's sexual desire, I'd discovered that the source of low libido is usually multilayered. It's psychological. It's relational. It's cultural. One biological theory I studied had a fatalistic component: Once we fulfill our reproductive purposes, desire is done. I didn't believe that. To me, desire is like a plant that needs the right care and conditions to stay alive.

A couple of weeks later I arrived at my office soaked. The failure of a flimsy three-dollar street umbrella that turned inside out had exposed me to the driving horizontal rain—and I was already harried from the subway ride. When I checked my voice mail, I had a message from Kasha. She wanted to know if I could fit her in for an emergency session.

She still wasn't a patient, but I needed some clarity on her commitment to Alex before I could consider suggesting formal couples counseling. I had an opening after lunch.

"I received an unmarked package this morning at my office," she told me. "Inside was this little black cocktail dress and a note telling me to meet in the lobby of the Four Seasons Hotel tonight at eight. There was no signature. I'm sure it's the Russian. What do I do?"

"What was your first reaction?"

"Anticipation. Excitement. I strutted around my office feeling superior to all the drones slaving away at their computers because I had a sexy secret. A powerful and mysterious man had summoned me for sex." Kasha was at her writerly best. "All day I've been fantasizing about what accessories to wear and how the evening will go."

"Yet you urgently had to see me today. Does that suggest part of you doesn't want to go? Tell me about that side of the conflict."

"I really do love Alex," she said, suddenly welling up with tears. "I started to feel guilty. He's everything I ever wanted. I enjoy his company and conversation. I feel so loved and adored by him. He's my best friend. I'm afraid of losing him."

"But you need passion, excitement, and adventure."

"That, too. We had it. I don't know what happened. I can't imagine life without that, so . . ." I sensed an imminent about-face. "So I'm thinking of leaving Alex."

"Those qualities are an important source of vitality," I

agreed. "The Russian awoke or reawoke that dormant part of you. And so powerfully that you're questioning a relationship that has already fulfilled you in so many ways."

"But the Russian is so fucking sexy," she said, and sighed. "Why can't I feel this way with Alex?"

Good question. Great question. I told Kasha to forget about Alex and the Russian for just a moment. I had the opening I'd been hoping for. Instead of looking for external sources to ignite her sexually, I asked what she had to give. "Can you take responsibility for cultivating your own sexual energy?"

"I *am* sexy," she insisted, as if my question was ridiculous.

"You *look* sexy," I said. "You can *act* sexy. But you are either passive—with Alex—or submissive—with the Russian. What do *you* want?" I told her this before. Would she hear it now?

Kasha still had no answer, and she looked to me, hoping I'd supply one. "You don't know because you're disconnected from your sensuality. That's what all this angst is trying to tell you."

"So what do I do?" Kasha whispered, still teary.

"Alex *could* be a safe base for you to start over and explore your erotic side. But you have to be able to tolerate the risk and uncertainty. You have to look inside yourself."

I believe that the four factors associated with sexual desire in the study mentioned earlier—distance, novelty, danger, and power—are all simply titillations, fleeting excitements, and, to cut to the heart of the matter, just a shot of dopamine in the reward center of the brain. They are fun to play with in moderation, and each comes with its own little hangover. All fire and no security eventually wears down desire as well.

Sex therapists have long worked to manipulate this balance of security versus fire when they assign homework. And patients have long complained that assignments such as planned dates and planned sex feel too scripted. They resist, or try once and abandon the effort. I value this instinct about inauthenticity because they've already felt stifled by their own sexual artifices. They want to be motivated to have sex spontaneously, and the solution is to be creative from an organic place. The important question is how does one get to that core, authentic place—particularly with all the cultural messages that we internalize?

Sexual desire isn't all about appearances, as Kasha liked to imagine. *Desire is energy.* Libido is a natural current that we all possess *internally*—and it is not reserved solely for the beautiful people, nor is it bestowed upon us by an external source like Aphrodite or a mysterious Russian man. Sometimes we only get a glimpse, but we all have it and we know it when we feel it or see it. Libido is a larger force than sex; it's what fuels all of our passions, creativity, and vitality. However, our visceral sexual sensations are fragile and can get easily constricted, ignored, or shut down by circumstances in our relationships, culture, or within ourselves. The result can be numbness or lack of sexual motivation.

I wanted to teach Kasha to cultivate her sexual energy, to start her own fire. Learning how to tap into oneself as a source of sexual energy is the foundation of lasting desire. A notable number of the women I've seen for low libido don't report any history of sexual trauma, active religious repression, or relationship discord; in these cases, the cause of low desire isn't some external trauma that has occurred. Rather it is a lack of sexual development. In the absence of affirmation for female sexual exploration and assertion, women like Kasha simply internalize the ideals of their lovers. I've discovered that lasting desire is a process much greater than the simple act of copulation, it's a journey of self-connection and self-development.

I'm reminded of the movie *Runaway Bride*. Julia Roberts's character always orders her eggs the same way as the guy she's with. Then she realizes she's never been authentic, which is part of why she always runs away. So eventually she cooks a whole assortment of egg dishes and sits down to taste them all and discover what *she* actually likes. That's starting from the beginning. This is what Kasha needed to do.

Kasha left, excited yet unsure about her assignation. Here's what she described to me afterward, in her usual lush detail.

That night, at precisely eight P.M., she arrived in the Four Seasons Hotel lobby. The glow of a massive chandelier highlighted her perfectly fit black cocktail dress, chin-length auburn hair, and smoky eyes. The opulently appointed room buzzed with chatter, and heads turned in Kasha's direction as she floated through the marble lobby scanning the crowd for the Russian. Suddenly she stopped, and the ambient noise faded, leaving only the sound of her pounding heart. There, at the bar he stood, casually, wearing a stylish black suit, martini in hand. But it wasn't the Russian.

"Very nice. I'm pleased," Alex said, as she approached. He handed her a room key. "I want you to go upstairs. I will join you shortly."

In the suite Kasha discovered on the bed a box containing lingerie. She unpacked it slowly, while collecting her thoughts. Alex, not the Russian. To her surprise she felt warm, a rush of joy and relief. She realized in that moment that her dalliance with the Russian was simply a substitute for what she really wanted from Alex. And from herself.

Kasha undressed, laid her clothes across an armchair, and slipped into the lingerie, fantasizing about what *she* wanted to do after Alex arrived.

When Kasha had left our session that afternoon, she was still ambivalent. The idea of cultivating her own eroticism was still vague and was largely overwhelmed by the dress she'd received and its pressing allusion to future excitement.

I did not know that Alex had sent the dress—until they told me the story when Alex came in for his next session. He brought Kasha with him. They were excited about their night together and wanted to share the details.

He had gone much farther with his homework assignment than instructed. He'd made a risky move. I'm not sure why I was so surprised. Alex was a very dedicated, studious patient. I wanted to give him a standing ovation. He'd had to dig deep, summon the sexual confidence of his fantasies, and embrace it. This isn't a skill I can teach; I can only guide someone in that direction. What Alex had done was a triumph of overcoming fear and finding his potential.

I was proud of them both.

And surprised that they never came to see me again.

Had they decided to terminate therapy prematurely, believing that one victory meant their work was done? Patients commonly make that mistake and set themselves up for disappointment. They quit when breakthroughs are made, but the energy and hopefulness they feel obscures the bumpy road ahead.

Alex and Kasha had one great night, but change, for most people, is a slow transformation. An assiduous uncovering. New thoughts and emotions eventually percolate upward and translate into action. Implementing new behavior is a painstaking process of practice and regression. Even though Alex and Kasha had tasted the potential to transform (and rekindle) their sexual relationship, I was skeptical and had no way to tell how long the aftereffects of their night at the Four Seasons would last.

Not because of Alex, though. He'd done his part. But I didn't believe I had been particularly effective with Kasha. In my brief time with her, she was defensive and competitive, and not willing to give up what worked for her in the immediate moment for the benefit of longer-term fulfillment. Kasha was intelligent, but her ability to self-reflect was poor, largely because she was a beautiful woman who lived in a bubble of easy adoration, unacquainted with the rewards that lay beyond the praise. And when the bubble popped . . . I expected it would be quite painful for her.

I also didn't trust that she would give up the Russian.

If I had any hope, it was that Alex and Kasha authentically valued their bond, and that that—along with incremental successes—would keep them on a forward path. Maybe their relationship would be one of those rare situations in psychotherapy when a rapid shift does occur. Maybe the night at the Four Seasons was a transformative catalyst. This kind of relationship crisis, with all of its disappointment and fears, can create a crucible so intense that one experience burns itself into the brain and crystallizes the kind of profound and lasting change that only love can propel us toward.

PAUL

A few months after opening my private practice, I came home one hot summer afternoon to an eviction notice on the front door, the electricity turned off, and my roommates all in a scramble. We discovered that our "landlord," Nestor, had illegally sublet the apartment to the eight of us, pocketed the cash, and disappeared. The owner of the building discovered us living there, accused us of squatting, shut off the electricity, and threatened to have the police curb our belongings by the next day. It was hot, dark, and total mayhem in the apartment when I walked in. I found it fascinating to watch the reactions people have to chaos. A few decided to throw a naked party. Sophie stole a bunch of my clothes and took off for Queens (I never heard from her again), and I, along with three others, grabbed the first apartment we could find on Craigslist. We landed just down the street from my practice—in the heart of Times Square.

Now this kind of haste didn't exactly situate us in a conventional apartment building. At street level was a rowdy Irish pub; a "massage" parlor took up the entire second floor, and my friends and I rented a flat that took up the whole third and final floor. Of note, our front door was on the second floor, right next to the "massage" parlor door. There were four of us, all women, and we were just happy to find a place, and elated to have our own rooms, even though the space was previously an office and the floors were covered by that cheap gray office carpet, reminding me that my bedroom was probably once a cubicle.

Despite the midtown location, this apartment was only convenient one day of the year: New Year's. We could go up on the roof and watch the ball of lights drop, and have some champagne just above the fray. Otherwise, carrying home my groceries through a morass of tourists with a constant upward gaze, transfixed by the sparkling billboard ads—a giant Planter's peanut, a giant Target logo—made me wonder why they came all the way from wherever to take snapshots of commercials. It was a veritable corporate parade, a Disneyland of banal consumer products in bright lights. I was constantly getting bumped, pushed, or just plain smacked around while people took photos of the giant M&M'S. Stepping outside my front door was like getting tossed inside of a washing machine.

Each day as I set out for work, I would see a massage parlor patron skulking down the hall on his way to his pleasures. The moment we passed each other was often awkward, filled with the tacit knowledge that we shared about where he was going and what he was about to do. The men usually hustled by, heads down, eyes on the hallway floor, while I tried to steal an inconspicuous glance at their faces, curious about what kind of man would patronize this type of sex service.

But no matter how many men I saw, I couldn't come up with any prototype for the customers. I encountered the young, the old, the handsome, and the homely. I saw business suits and work shirts. I watched a United Nations parade of men—from Indians to Hasidic Jews. I wondered how many of them were husbands and boyfriends, and if their wives and girlfriends had any clue about these visits.

Sometimes my flat mates and I would try to peek inside the massage parlor when the opaque door cracked open and a middle-aged Korean woman greeted her customers with a demure smile. Now and then we'd even invent mischievous reasons to knock ourselves, like borrowing paper towels or scissors. Once I tried to get a massage but was told, "No massage for ladies."

We still found ways to have fun with the massage parlor. The speaker on the call box that visitors buzzed to get into our building was so loud that whatever we said at our end was broadcast to anyone passing by on 47th Street. Each time the buzzer went off, we hoped it would be one of our many friends dropping in, but we could just as easily say "Hello?" only to hear someone respond, "Massage?" Oops, sorry. Wrong button.

Too often the call box buzzed late into the night. As payback, one of us might yell into the intercom, "If you're looking for a blow job, press number two!"—knowing full well that anyone still on the street could hear. It seemed funny, and an easy shot to take.

One evening, on my way out, a well-marinated pub-goer stumbled up the stairs into the second-floor hallway and urinated on the hardwood floor. The Korean woman emerged with a bucket of water and we cleaned in amiable silence, her English conveniently nonexistent. I carefully observed her heavily made-up face and outdated, cheap, sexy clothing that looked like it came from one of the sex shops in Hell's Kitchen. I thought to myself, Is this what men want?

One answer to my question was Paul, a recently married bank executive in his early forties. A blustery alpha male, Paul strode into my office for his first appointment and, unlike most patients who wait for me to begin, zoomed right past the standard pleasantries and started firing words at me at a machine-gun pace, even before he sat down. "This is my problem," he said, in a raspy voice. "I'm not having sex with my wife. I'm having trouble keeping it up. So I'm having sex with prostitutes. I'll give you five sessions to fix this."

"You have a time limit?"

"I'm not one of those people who like to lie on a couch and talk every week."

I wasn't sure how I was going to create a bond with this guy. An important part of psychotherapy is the relationship, which takes time to develop, and he was basically trying to get help while bypassing the relationship. Paul made direct eye contact—though it felt like he was looking through me. He related to me in that way one does when ordering around a server in a restaurant—without any respect for that person as another human, as if I were simply some entity there for his service. This interaction can't be that different from prostitution for him, I thought; an intimate situation with no intimacy.

"Let's talk about your fee," he snapped.

"We discussed this on the phone," I said. "It's one hundred and fifty dollars an hour."

"Too much."

I knew that Paul could well afford me. But money wasn't really the point. He seemed to be making a power grab.

"You're really trying to take charge here," I said.

Paul shrugged. "*I'm* paying for the therapy."

Paul was obviously comfortable with the arrogant and entitled control he assumed over women he paid. I couldn't let him stay in that position.

"Yes, you *are* paying for therapy," I agreed. "What does that mean to you?"

His answer was an attack. "How much experience do you have again, Doc?"

Paul's hit landed right on my weak spot and I was starting to chafe. In order to continue, I tried to imagine a poor suffering man behind this puffery. "You're here for help," I said. "I give you credit for showing up. You could have gone to a prostitute. But listen, Paul, instead of questioning my value, try and think of being here as making an investment in yourself and your marriage. Seeking treatment is really an indicator of how much you value *yourself*." I let that resonate.

"And, in any case, you will *not* pay me less than a prostitute," I said, smiling, even as I realized they probably made more than I did.

Paul mulled that over. "Okay, Doc," he said, as if the whole interchange had been meaningless. "We can keep your rate. Now let's get down to business."

"Good. I'm glad you chose to see me," I said, trying to imagine how he related to the women in his life. "I will do my best to help you."Paul described how he sometimes ordered women on an outcall basis to service him in the back of a limo while he drove around making business calls, as well as frequent visits to massage parlors. Ooooh! . . . massage parlors, the mysterious massage parlor—I couldn't wait to hear all about the appeal of the parlor ladies. I rarely saw them going in and out, only their patrons. I wondered about their exotic beauty. However, Paul was most interested in talking about the impotence he experienced with his wife, so I made a mental note to ask about parlor life later.

"How long have you been having an erection problem?" I asked.

"Off and on, ever since I met her. I need tons of stimulation and sometimes I still lose my hard-on halfway through. I'm amazed she married me anyway."

"How does your wife—what's her name?—react?"

"Claire gets pissed off, obviously. She thinks I'm not attracted to her, which is really not true. I just don't *feel* that much pleasure during sex. My dick goes . . . almost numb."

"But you *are* attracted to her?"

"Yes. Very much. She's got that short, petite, curvy body type that I love."

So what's the problem? He loves her, he finds her attractive, yet he can't maintain an erection? Before I could formulate a solid hypothesis I needed to consider Paul's age, medical condition, and stress level—all factors that can contribute to erectile dysfunction. Paul didn't have any extenuating medical problems, and although it is more likely for a forty-year-old man to need extra stimulation than for an eighteen-year-old, Paul's dysfunction was specific to committed relationships. This indicated a psychological genesis.

I also needed to know more about Claire. Paul said they'd been married for eight months, and although she had a strong personality and gave him "a lot of shit," he liked it. "I guess some men would find her intimidating, but I think she's challenging and exciting. A great match for me. I like a woman I can feel a little threatened by; she keeps me on my toes. We're both competitive and can get into power struggles."

"Can you describe her sexually?"

Paul's eyes lit up. "She loves sex. I think she has a bigger sex drive than I do."

"Who initiates?"

"Mostly Claire. She tells me what she wants in bed. She doesn't hold back. I like that about her . . ."

"But?" I wanted Paul to finish his thought.

"But, like I said, she gets mad when I lose my erection."

"What is that like for you?"

"Terrible. She gets hostile."

"How?"

"She asks me what my problem is and then she gets all weepy and thinks I don't want her anymore."

Who initiates sex is a loaded issue. It brings up a bunch of questions all at once: Am I desirable? Am I loved or not? Who is needier? Who has more emotional control? Sometimes when a woman initiates sex, a man can feel acute anxiety about getting an erection. I asked him what he'd done to address this erection issue.

"I started taking Viagra without her knowing," he said, dialing down his rapid-fire responses a notch. "But I don't like the idea of taking pills for what should happen naturally with my wife."

When I reflected that statement back to Paul, saying that it seemed as if he felt a lot of pressure about keeping his erection, he enthusiastically agreed. "That's all I can think about during sex. I'm constantly in my head, worrying, What if I lose this hard-on again?"

"So you don't enjoy sex with Claire, even though you desperately want to."

"I get most of my pleasure when *she's* satisfied," he said. "But I get stressed about it."

"And this happens *only* with your wife—not the prostitutes?"

"Yes. Actually, I *have* had this problem in some of my previous serious relationships," he said, with a sudden frown.

Erectile dysfunction, variously put as "I can't get it up" or "I can't feel anything in my penis" or "I have a beautiful girlfriend, but . . ." was the most common of the complaints I'd begun hearing from men of all ages. In fact, the situation seems almost epidemic and, curiously, more often has a primarily psychological (not medical) genesis. Viagra and similar medications have become fashionable, including in the club scene, where young guys who don't need chemical assistance carry a pill for insurance, along with a condom, when they go out, in case they hook up.

But Paul's erectile dysfunction was situational. He could get consistent erections, only not with Claire. "I'm fine when I masturbate," Paul said. "Or when I go to massage parlors. In fact, I get much more pleasure out of sex then."

"Tell me what you like about the massage parlor experience."

"There is no pressure at all. I don't care about those girls. I pay them to satisfy me; usually blow jobs or hand jobs. I like to hire two at a time, have them pull their tops down and I fondle them while they take turns touching and sucking on me. It's much more erotic for me, and the best part is that I don't have to think about their pleasure. They are like nonbeings."

I wrote the word "nonbeings" in my notebook. Once again, I was faced with a client's distasteful attitude. I wondered why I—why does *any* woman—bother working out, and spending God knows how much money on expensive makeup, and perfect highlights for our hair, when a man like Paul, with a beautiful wife, can only get it up with a lady who buys 1980s-style black latex leggings with holes in them from the sex shop on 48th Street? Do women really not know some essential truth about what men want? Do we refuse to accept what's staring us in the face? Something to consider, I thought, as I scheduled another appointment for Paul.

Listening to men talk about women, which gave me access to a hidden cache of information about what they really want, what they find sexy or beautiful, wasn't what I'd thought it would be, and I found my own psyche threatened and a bit overwhelmed by their appraisals.

One comment that I never get used to is, "My wife has gained weight and I'm not attracted to her anymore." These men are totally indignant about it, too, and some use their displeasure to justify cheating, or they avoid sex, while silently simmering with resentment. One patient of mine separated from his wife and then made it a condition that she lose weight before he was willing move back into the house.

Then I would meet these wives who had supposedly committed the egregious insult of gaining weight, only to usually discover it was no more than twenty pounds. I understand that men are visual, but is some extra flesh on a woman's body really such an affront?

When I dug deeper, I was usually heartened to discover that many of these men felt put off by wives and girlfriends who'd "let themselves go" because they feared that it really meant these women had lost interest in *them* sexually. So the men's anger wasn't based simply on how their women *looked,* on how they didn't labor to conform to cultural clichés of attractiveness. The weight gain was a metaphor for direct rejection, a materialized message that the man was undesirable, not worth staying in shape for, and even that the woman might not care about him anymore.

Perhaps counterintuitively for our culture, in my experience men's desire is not *completely linked* to a woman's specific body measurements. When I ask men to describe the qualities of the women they are most attracted to, or their most beguiling lovers, they will of course often talk about their beauty. And when I get them to elaborate on what exactly is beautiful, they will narrow it down to certain physical attributes at first, but what breaks through in the final analysis is that what they find most alluring is this: a woman who views herself as a sexual being, enjoys her sexuality, and is willing to express it.

I noticed during my postgraduate work with a hospital crisis team in Brooklyn that the same curvy female body type evoked a very different response on the other side of the bridge. Each day I drove through the Brooklyn streets in a van with three men:

one Dominican, one Puerto Rican, and one from Trinidad. They all loved to stare out the windows and admire the Latina and African-American ladies, women with thick thighs harnessed by tight jeans, their abundant bodies joyfully spilling out of their intentionally tiny clothes. My companions leered with appreciation and excitement. Okay, they practically frothed and panted like hungry animals. And even though I had been socialized to a completely different beauty standard, I couldn't help but recognize these women's sex appeal myself.

These ladies *were* sexy. And they understood something important: It was all in the way they carried their bodies. It was as if they were saying, "I know you want me and I totally love that." They owned their physicality with the pride of a man who takes his fancy, polished new car out for a drive, just to show it off to the neighborhood. These ladies took their time to carefully display every curve, boasting and taunting with each slow, swaggering step. I saw one Latina, who may have been in her later middle-aged years, just swinging down the boulevard in her tight pants, high heels, and a little ruffled top decorated with brightly colored flowers. Her shoulders were back and her head high; she made eye contact and had an easy smile. She walked as if she was flirting with the world, a celebration of femininity, an ode to life.

Caucasian culture has been subjected to some pretty powerful social conditioning about thinness, which made it difficult for some of my patients to look with approval at the women in their lives who varied from it. These three gawking female appreciators I worked with in Brooklyn seemed somehow more liberated in their sexuality than some of the men on my couch with all of their conditions placed on their partner's attractiveness.

Most men, however, know that true sexiness is much greater than good looks while women often make the mistake of confusing beauty with sexiness. For men, sexiness is beauty. I think that's good news for a woman. *Sexiness is to show interest in sex.* Therefore it's a choice, a behavior, and not solely some mandate on your physical dimensions.

One of my patients, a slight and soft-spoken Quaker man married for twenty-five years, put it to me like this: "I want to try having sex doggy-style with my wife and she refuses to do it. She says her butt is too big and she doesn't want me to look at it. To be honest, I don't care about the size of her ass. I love my wife. I just want her to have fun with me!"

This is what men want.

At Paul's next session, I picked up where we'd left off, as per my notes. "So you think of the women you hire to pleasure you as nonbeings," I reminded him. "That's very different from the way you describe Claire, who is strong and challenging." I let my tone border on the reproachful. "What's the erotic appeal of these women who somehow don't count?"

"I'd never be interested in them romantically," he said. "They're unattractive, passive and submissive, so I can give them all kinds of orders and they will do just about anything. I don't do anything to harm them, but I like to put them in positions where they are slightly exposed and vulnerable while they service me."

"But you don't do this with Claire," I said. "Only women whom you consider inferior."

"Yes, and that is precisely the turn-on."

Paul was getting off on the act of debasement. Subjugating these "inferior nonbeings" liberated Paul from the performance anxiety that he experienced with his wife and allowed him to feel superior. I'd been right about the subtext of Paul's initial approach to me and the other women he paid: He needed to create a hierarchy right away.

Performance anxiety is a jargon word for the very common and erection-destroying phenomenon of being so focused on one's sexual performance that one freezes. This blow to sexual potency can be humiliating, especially when it happens repeatedly and, at worst, with someone you want to impress—which is when it's most likely to happen. However, I had a hard time sympathizing with Paul's performance anxiety while he trumpeted the delights of violating women. As a woman, it was difficult for me to listen to Paul and other men describe how they're able to feel better about themselves by depreciating a woman. I was disheartened that men wanted to do this. What did this mean about men? I wished that I could have explained it away by looking at Paul as an anomaly. But, truth be told, Paul was not atypical, sexually deviant, or creepy. He was an everyday guy who felt love for his wife. I noticed among my other patients that many of the men who were visiting massage parlors did have some sort of sexual dysfunction or at the very least a sexual anxiety of sorts with the women that they were actually interested in. Maybe what disturbed me the most was that dehumanization and degradation seemed to be a pervasive source of sexual arousal for these men.

Just the week before, I'd walked into my apartment building to find the police in the second-floor hallway, raiding the massage parlor, shouting, "Get up. Get your clothes on!"

I tried to unlock our apartment door quickly and duck inside, but an officer approached and asked if he could search my place for girls who had fled. I didn't think anyone could have gotten in, but I let him look anyway.

He checked the premises and left. Several hours later, after dinner in the kitchen with friends, I went to the bathroom and discovered a teenaged Asian girl hiding in our shower. She looked frightened and kept saying, "Help me," in a thick accent. I went to grab my cell phone, and she ran off through the apartment and scurried out the front door.

I still have no idea how she'd gotten in. Was she some kind of ninja? A trapdoor in the parlor ceiling? Spiderwoman ability to climb the outside walls and balance on a ledge? Or maybe she just jimmied our lock. I was worried that she had been trafficked, and her terrified young face haunted me. The next day a giant fruit basket appeared by our front door with a note: "You are friend now." Great, be careful what you wish for, I thought.

Every day I had to walk through some part of Times Square to get home. Mayor Giuliani had given the area a big makeover, but Times Square was still teeming with services to satisfy sexual needs, especially marketed toward men in the midtown finance industry. One evening, I was in a lounge frequented by Wall Street types and tourists and was approached by an elegant woman representing a high-end escort service. To my surprise, she offered me a job. I was chagrined. What did I look like to her? I'm a doctor, not a prostitute, I thought and bristled. Yet I was also a bit flattered that she thought I was a "model-quality escort," and her proposition made me realize that call girl services are literally camped all around Times Square, all competing for the same target: men with money. Hunting, circling, and ensnaring. In-service, out-call, massage, models, Asian, Russian, Brazilian, high-end, trashy, young, illegal, etc. At work and at home, the sex service industry swirled around me.

To answer the question I posed earlier: Is *this* what men want? Some of them, yes. But I don't mean just the anonymous sex or cheaply dressed pleasure-givers. What these men *want* is to have an emotional craving sated in a cheap and easy way. It's not simply sexual, it's emotional.

I've often thought that massage parlor menus should read:

Services:

Special #1: Feel important.

Special #2: Feel powerful.

Special # 3: Get nurturing and soothing.

This would more accurately define the expensive role-play they engage in. For one hour, these men can direct their very own personal drama, acting out the gratification of their deepest longings and frustrations. Yes, right there, in the heart of the theater district, the remedy for their greatest psychological vulnerabilities, sold as a commodity, advertised by flashing pink lights, and dispensed by those who couldn't care less about them. The problem with this interaction is that they are not really solving their issues; they are pretending for an hour and then walking off with the same emotional deficits with which they arrived, and adding to that a real disconnect in their relationships.

How did I end up in the middle of all of this? I wondered. I was losing perspective on men, becoming disoriented. You might believe that a sex therapist would quickly become desensitized to hearing stories of men cheating. But at the time, they made me quite uncomfortable. The more tales of infidelity I heard, the more my anxiety built. Sometimes the man across from me would suddenly go blurry, his words falling on deaf ears as I withdrew into my personal worries.

At times, in session, I felt as if I had lived a pampered and sheltered life and someone had taken me to the scariest section of Skid Row and left me there. I would have preferred my old wonderful world of denial and fantasy, where I could hold hands with my lover and skip through sunny fields of romance. Yet I couldn't escape—this was my job. I was now forced to look directly at the ugly, disfigured side of human relating: Yes, at times men want to exploit women, harm them, cheat on them, use them like a piece of meat. The confluence of my experiences with Rami and his friends, and my patients, led to the aggressive penetration of all of my fantasies and high ideals. This rupture of my grand bubble was painful. It was also an opportunity to mature.

I knew I had to find some new way of thinking that could integrate into my belief system everything I'd been learning. I was going to have to overcome my judgment and fear or transfer these patients to new therapists. My strategy, and my struggle, was to remain the detached scientific observer, seeking to explore, taking notes, and trying to understand. I also reminded myself not to generalize: Not all men were like the men I was treating. I had known plenty of great men in my life. I had to hold on to that thought and those memories.

I reflected on the young girl hiding in my shower, trembling, unsure if she was safer with me or out in the street, and I thought about how these sex services weren't just some innocuous enjoyment in life, but something that did real harm. I became determined to effect change upon this world I had entered. This exploitation fantasy Paul had was big business, and clearly there was ample supply and demand. I decided that my role was to intervene on the side of the demand. Sometimes I was amused that, as a therapist, I was actually competing with the sex services. What made some of these guys choose me? How could I compete with the instant gratification, the fantasy they sought, the limitless menu of beautiful women? Some men went to a brothel. Others came to me. But I was a different kind of madam. I wasn't the distraction these men were looking for. I was not a purveyor of pleasure, but rather a purveyor of truth. I gave them exactly what they didn't want, but I gave them what they needed.

Paul always came in for sessions after he got off of work, and he frequently asked me to push the limit on how late I wanted to stay. One evening, he arrived visibly stressed. He marched in, sat down, and as was his habit, began talking immediately, not pausing, not seeking my input.

"I think my company's going through a financial crisis," he said. "The media has started investigating our firm." Paul's tone was foreboding, and anything but sober. He was tense and distracted, his eyes darting as he got lost in his head. I allowed him the catharsis of relieving his stress, which took much of the session. But even though he spoke passionately, I felt estranged. We had no real bond. It was as if I were a faceless body onto which he could dump his pain. I wondered if his wife ever sensed this disconnection.

"How are you managing the stress?" I asked.

"I mostly spend long hours at the office—though I did call an escort service again at lunch today," he said, tepidly. Paul's visits to massage parlors had increased as he continued to feel overwhelmed at work.

"Am I picking up on some guilt from you tonight?" I asked.

"Yes. Claire would be devastated if she knew. I really adore her. I just wish I got more pleasure from our sex life."

"Instead, you've found a sexual supplement."

"I guess I've just rationalized that I will always need one," he said, resigned. "It's not that big of a deal, though. A lot of my friends think this way."

Again with the casual attitude toward sexual relief outside of marriage—particularly a marriage that Paul wanted to stay in. He acted as if it was common for men to choose to get married *knowing* that they will eventually need or want a "sexual supplement."

Paul having sex outside of his marriage made no emotional sense to me. I didn't understand how he could believe he *loved* his wife. But apparently Paul could. And did. And he wasn't the first patient who'd made this claim. Even the sweet guy-next-door types whom you'd never suspect had an unfaithful bone in their bodies had confessed the same while sitting on my couch, leaving me to think, Oh, no. Not you, too? I had always believed that if a man was truly in love, he wouldn't seek sex elsewhere. If he did, then he couldn't *really* be in love. To me, love and fidelity went hand in hand.

If I had discovered that Rami had strayed, my first thought would have been that he didn't love me anymore. In fact, given the miles that separated us, and our history, not to mention Rami's gregarious personality, I often worried about what might be going on—especially now that I was listening to men all day and learning that being in love was *not* an insurance policy against infidelity. Could I, or any woman, ever trust a man?

As patients discussed their sexual motivations with me, I kept wondering what made a man act on the impulse—especially the men who said that love had nothing to do with cheating, that they remained crazy about their wives and lovers. Were there identifiable emotional patterns or personality traits associated with unfaithfulness?

I looked for reasons beyond the obvious—you know: If he's done it before or if he did it with you, then he is a cheater by definition. I also checked in with any women I could engage in this conversation, to get a sense of their experiences. The general consensus ranged from these men having a lack of moral character, to the excuse men often fall back on: It's biological. Men are just built to spread their seed.

But that conclusion seemed too easy, too knee-jerk, especially when one factored in the more complex emotional, social, and psychological layers.

I wanted to see what the core motivation was for Paul. What did he *really* get out of unpressured sex on the side besides a hard-on and an orgasm? Was that the whole point? Or was he avoiding something with Claire, and himself? Paul had compartmentalized his wife and the prostitutes, but it didn't look like the hackneyed virgin/whore complex. Paul said Claire loved sex and was the initiator in their intimate encounters. She was clearly no virgin.

I asked Paul to tell me in detail about his most recent sexual experience with Claire. "Last night, we were in bed and she started by kissing my neck and rubbing my crotch," he said, matter-of-factly.

"How was that for you?"

"Truth? Her desire felt like a demand and I can't get hard that fast. I wish she would let me initiate sex."

"You could."

"Yes, but honestly, sometimes I want to avoid her. Like I said, I start worrying that I'm going to lose my erection and her getting mad about it. Anyways, I don't want to reject her, so I go right into a fantasy in order to get hard. Last night, I thought about this pretty young girl at the massage parlor who gave me a hand job while I put my hand inside her skirt. It turned me on that she didn't ask me to touch her and was probably too passive or maybe afraid to ask me to stop."

What Paul said really challenged the notion that guys always want sex at any time with anyone, and revealed that, in fact, even for men conditions need to be right.

"And that worked for you?"

"I had to turn Claire over on her belly so I didn't have to look into her eyes and could keep the fantasy going. She likes that position anyway, and I can just wrap my hand around her body and touch her. She gets off so easy, thank God."

Paul had just wanted to get through the sexual experience without failing, and in order for that to happen, he had to completely check out. Yet despite what he'd told me about how much he loved Claire, I saw no trace of that love during the sex.

"I didn't think of it that way," he said, when I shared my assessment. "I just want to get an erection and please her. I try to give her orgasms."

"You're making your erection and her satisfaction more important than really connecting with Claire."

"Well, my erection *is* important or we can't have sex."

I would have loved to have had Claire in the office to describe her experience of their sex life. I imagined it would be much different than what Paul might believe. However, Paul, like many men who came to see me, didn't want his wife to know he was seeking treatment.

"You talk a lot about giving her pleasure, but you sound pretty self-focused," I said. "The sex you're describing seems more anxious than erotic. I understand why you do it, but you're off in your head, a spectator, fantasizing. You can't relax and let Claire please you like the girls at the massage parlor because you don't think of her as a nonbeing. So to compensate, you focus on your penis and her orgasm."

"Otherwise she gets angry."

"And how do you feel about that?"

He chuckled at the cliché therapeutic question.

"I really want you to answer that," I insisted. "With a *feeling* word."

"Humiliated. Inadequate." Paul stared at a spot on the carpet. "Of course I want to avoid those feelings."

"Why?"

"I'm terrified of not being good enough for Claire—and then rejected." I didn't know why Paul had suddenly revealed such a primitive fear aloud, but I was glad he had, instead of letting it lurk just below the surface of his usual bravado. Paul twisted uncomfortably in his seat.

I softened toward Paul for a moment, and my eyes moistened as I could sense a real pain in him. I noticed that as he looked down, his knee was shaking. I could tell that my reaction made him nervous, and he began to shut down. It was a counterintuitive moment. I was at my most compassionate, yet that made Paul feel vulnerable, which caused him to feel threatened. He became quiet. I paused for a moment, then decided to move in on his anxiety.

"What are you feeling right now Paul?"

"Uneasy."

"You're starting to let me know you on a deeper level. Is that making you anxious?"

"I didn't say anxious, I said *uneasy,*" he snapped.

"Okay, uneasy. I want to understand *exactly* what you're feeling."

"Fine. I'm anxious, I'm getting that same feeling I get when I'm around my wife. I don't want you to see my weakness."

"Yet I can see it and you want to attack and you want to hide."

"I hate these analyses, they feel like criticism."

"You are being really brave to talk about this with me. I feel much closer to you, and I would never want to reject you for sharing yourself."

He simply looked down, and our session had come to an end. Paul was making progress, but he couldn't stand my mirroring; to him, my observations were reflections of his imperfection. My attempts at knowing Paul were intolerable for him. And there was something else: I had fended off his attempts to minimize me, and now he saw me in a position to judge him, and this elicited a familiar anxiety response, causing him to be impotent with me. I had an epiphany. I had been so busy freaking out about all of Paul's extramarital excursions that I had lost focus and almost missed the underlying problem: his vulnerability. The performance anxiety was just a symptom.

The more I thought about it, the more I realized that what bothered me most about Paul was that he was willing to settle for the easy way out. He was avoiding performance anxiety with an excessive focus on his wife's pleasure. He was using giving to avoid the anxiety of receiving. Having a sense of entitlement about receiving pleasure is a reflection of one's core self-worth. With prostitutes Paul was attempting to reclaim his sense of self, and along with it his belief in his right to receive pleasure. At home, Paul was too busy trying to cover up his anxiety, and it was blocking his enjoyment of his wife.

The result of all of these compensations for Paul and Claire was total disconnection.

Sex services, like the massage parlor in my building, were a common attempt to resolve this alienation. I've even known men who, out of that loneliness that comes from an estranged society, spend every evening in a Hooters or a strip club and try and get to know the women who work there, pretending they are actual friends.

I wanted Paul to consider sharing his concerns about his work situation with Claire. It might lay the groundwork for a more intimate conversation down the line.

"I don't like to talk about work with my wife," he said.

"What makes that difficult?"

"I was raised middle-class and worked my way up to the position I have now," Paul explained. "Claire comes from old money and her family has never really accepted me. They still make me feel like an outsider. They even force her to keep her trust money in a separate account that I don't have access to. I've worked hard to prove myself to Claire and to her family, but with my business in danger of collapsing financially I don't want to let her see how that worries me."

"What exactly are you trying to prove?"

"Her parents had someone else in mind for her to marry, but she picked me. I've always wondered if I measure up, I guess. I want to prove that they can accept me. That she can accept me. That I'm okay. I don't want her to regret that she chose me."

"So you've never felt the equal of Claire or her family?"

"No. She's so accomplished, sharp. Her whole family is like that. Believe it or not, as loud as I am, I'm the quiet one at her family gatherings. I shut down. It's like I'm in a competition and I can't win. It's the worst freakin' feeling."

Paul lumbered through his words as if each one was painful to admit, even to himself.

"And so you feel obligated to project an image of success both at work—and in bed." I could see on Paul's face that he made the connection.

"I *am* very successful," he replied, defensively.

"Yes, you're successful, but there's a cost. When you're stressed, like you are now, you choose to pull away from Claire, and that doesn't seem to be helping you."

"That's why I use call girls." He seemed to deflate, exhausted.

"Yes, and that's also why you can't keep an erection with Claire. You've created a phony perfect persona to hide parts of yourself from your wife and her family—and you suspect they see right through you anyway. But rather than help matters, you withdraw and end up more isolated, and feel bad. The result is more pressure for you when you're with Claire or her family.

"I can see that being a part of the family is important to you, but you're trying so hard to overcome your perceived inadequacies and be accepted that you're wearing yourself out."

Paul put his head down.

"You don't want to constantly have to prove yourself," I added, tenderly. "You want unconditional love. You're so proud to be married to Claire; you love her and you're scared that somehow you will be exposed as not good enough—and that she will stop loving you."

He nodded.

"Do you love Claire, Paul?"

He nodded again.

"Say it out loud."

"I love my wife."

Tears.

"Right now, you're being driven by the fear instead of love," I said. "We need to turn that around. Love your wife. If you want to be a good husband, there needs to be intimacy. Let her see you, Paul. Let her know you."

Finally, he sat silently and listened to me. I felt myself wanting to encourage him, felt my heart really warming to this man.

I also understood how I had gotten lost in my initial reaction of fear when listening to the stories of my patients. Upset by the need of some men to cheat, or to put women in abject positions, I'd formed negative conclusions and made generalizations. I needed to detach a bit and remember that it's very easy to get focused on how "bad" behavior is, make moral judgments, label men pejoratively, and believe that this is simply male nature, and that's that.

As Paul opened up, he helped me to come out of that haze, and I could see that the sexual interactions with both his wife and the sex workers revealed a very important truth: Women are incredibly powerful to men. In fact, women are so powerful that it's overwhelming. Men need women to survive emotionally: our approval, our support, and our encouragement, all of which enables them to flourish in the world, to feel confident. Women's nurturing and comfort help the men in their lives to feel safe and grounded. All the women in Paul's life were powerful figures. He idealized his wife so much that he felt small. He devalued the sex workers so much that he felt large. And he lost all measure of himself in their wake.

His issues had little to do with sex. It wasn't about simple sexual taste or a man's natural need for a sexual supplement. Instead it had everything to do with Paul's sense of self and his ability to hold on to his self-worth in the presence of the woman he loved. This is important because this is where the hope in this story lies. This is where the answers to my question "What do men want?" actually resides.

Paul wanted to love his wife and himself at the same time, and he needed her love desperately. I wanted to help Paul find that love and hold on to it, so he could be present with Claire.

Between Paul and the others I'd treated, I had started to notice a theme. Vulnerability. All these men seemed caught between their need for love and their fear of love. They reacted by creating these bizarre relationships and sexual approximations, then twisted and distorted them into substitutes for love—

pleasure-seeking, ego gratification, or fantastical romance—to get their needs met and still stay safe. They'd come to me claiming that they were in love, or wanted to be in love, but what they had was not even close. These guys were running away from the real thing. They needed to reexamine their definitions of love.

We all love the feeling of love, that warm euphoric state, but love is not simply one feeling. Nor is it easy. Along with the joy comes difficult emotions like anger, boredom, hurt. Then there is the formidable and inevitable avalanche of fear: of rejection, of disappointment, of losing yourself, of abandonment, of being found out as really unlovable. These fears can be irrational, but they can also come true.

Loving is more than just feelings. It's a skill. These guys seemed to be taking the easy way out. David (from Chapter One) wanted to be desired. Paul wanted power. Others want safety. I couldn't believe all these men sitting in front of me were focusing on what they were getting and not getting, and not thinking about what they were giving.

Nobody wanted to take a risk.

I wanted Paul to stop pulling away from Claire, to stop seeking solutions outside their marriage, and to move toward her instead. Paul was finally willing to try anything I suggested.

"I have a homework assignment for you," I said, checking the clock to make sure we had enough time left for me to explain.

Homework is the cornerstone of sex therapy. Patients are often assigned various sexual exercises designed to reprogram their sexual responses. Most male sexual functioning is simply reflex and can be retrained. Paul's erection was associated with self-consciousness, and I needed to get that reconditioned to a relaxed sensuality.

"Your assignment is to avoid an erection," I said. He looked surprised, but pressure of performance was the last thing I wanted him preoccupied with. "If you happen to get one, you're not allowed to seek an orgasm. You're also forbidden from trying to give Claire an orgasm. In fact, stay away from her genitals." I wanted him to try and be present in the moment. "Instead," I continued, "I want you to focus on just touching the rest of her body. Take your time and really try to feel her with your touch. Focus on your love for her with each of your senses. I want you to smell her, taste her, and really look at this woman you love, and appreciate what you see. Look into her eyes, kiss her slowly. Soulfully. When she touches you, do not think about your erection, just notice any sensation of pleasure and enjoy it—but do not act upon it. Stay with your right to feel pleasure, that same sense of entitlement that you have at the massage parlor.

"And I want you to initiate this *tonight* when you get home." Paul took it all in, seeming both uncertain yet determined, as was his nature, to complete the assignment successfully. "And I will see you next week and you can let me know how it went."

I left my office, dragging my rolling suitcase, and searched for a cab. I was on my way to the airport to catch a flight to Florida to see Rami. Some days I really wanted Rami to get a divorce; on other days, I rationalized it away, thinking that I didn't want marriage or kids and was happy with an unconventional relationship. Of course, trust issues lay at the bottom of it all, and I was still trying to work that out, still trying to not be afraid that leaving—or staying—would be a mistake.

Unfortunately, Friday evening is an impossible time to get a ride in Midtown. Desperate, I spotted a cab with its lights off, sitting at a traffic light. I knocked on the passenger side, and a hard-faced Indian man looked out and cracked the window.

"I'm off," he shouted.

"I know," I said. "But if you're going home and you live in Queens or Brooklyn, can you drop me off at LaGuardia?"

He thought for a moment.

"Please. I'm trying to go see my boyfriend!"

More thinking and the light was about to turn.

"Do it for love!" I said with a smile. Given his expression, love did not seem part of his vocabulary—at least at the moment.

"All right," I shouted. "I'll pay you sixty dollars."

"You're killing me," he said, but he let me in. He turned off the meter and hit the gas.

I had a habit of talking to cabdrivers about my romantic affairs, my existential crises, everything. And to my surprise, they often listened with voyeuristic pleasure and gave earnest advice. One even read my palm. I looked forward to seeing Rami, but Paul had wound me up and I needed to process my thoughts. I was uncomfortable sharing my personal neuroses even with my friends. I guess I feared they would think "And she's a psychologist?" as if a therapist should be able to manage her own problems. The anonymity of being a cab passenger allowed me to open up and tell my stories.

However, the irony didn't escape me. Like Paul, instead of being authentic and vulnerable in my own close relationships, I was using anonymous surrogates to meet my emotional needs. Even I couldn't avoid the instant gratification of the artificial connection.

I didn't think this driver would be receptive. When I peeked at his reflection in the rearview mirror, I could tell that he still wore his hard face. I sat in the corner of the backseat, diagonally from him, looking out at the skyline rushing—and sometimes crawling—by. But before long I grew uncomfortable with the impersonal silence. I slid over to the mid-floor hump, stuck my face close to the glass, and read his license.

"How are you this evening, Mohinder?" I said.

"Tired."

"What's it like being a cabdriver? You must have some pretty interesting conversations."

"Yes. Once, a woman even had a baby in the backseat."

"Wow."

"Where are you rushing to?" he asked.

"To Florida, to see my boyfriend. We visit each other on weekends."

"That sounds difficult."

Now it was my turn to be thoughtful. "Actually, I like it. But he wants me to move back to Florida and live with him."

"Will you?"

"He's still married. So why should I?"

"That doesn't make any sense. He's still married and he wants you to move in with him and his wife?"

I chuckled. "No, they've been separated for years. They don't even live in the same state."

"Ah. That works well for him, doesn't it? Perhaps he is afraid of commitment."

"No, I don't think so," I said, although I knew my self-deception was probably very easy to read.

"Oh? Well, I know how you can test him."

"How?" I wasn't sure I really wanted to know the answer.

"Simple. Just tell him that you are ready to move in right away and see what he does."

Mohinder was right. But I was afraid to do that. Didn't want to do that. Maybe later. Maybe.

As we finally neared the airport, I thought about Paul and how we all play games with intimacy. We move in close, then move away, opening and closing rhythmically, like a jellyfish expanding and contracting as it glides through the ocean. With humans, both partners do this dance, and if they're lucky, they achieve some sort of harmony. Paul was so busy trying to be the perfect husband, the perfect provider, the perfect penis, but he was never very authentic with Claire. I wondered how that worked for her.

Paul didn't wait until our next session to report in. He booked an emergency appointment the day I returned from Florida, charged into my office, and confronted me.

"What the hell am I paying you for?" he barked. Paul dropped to the couch and leaned close. "I get more help from the massage parlor!" he snarled.

Paul complained that my homework assignment had backfired. "I went home after our session," Paul explained. "Claire was already in bed reading a book. I took the book from her hands and set it on the nightstand. I grabbed her by the waist and pulled her body in close to mine. Remembering what you told me, I started by looking at her intently. Her body, her face, I wanted to really see them. I touched her cheek and told her how much I loved her. I said I loved every inch of her body—her breasts, her long legs, her flat stomach, her pussy, her toes, her eyes. Her mouth. I kept running my hands over her—and while I did this *I felt nothing*. I got no erection. I was just numb."

"Paul, the point was for you to *forget* about getting an erection. If it didn't happen, that's not a bad outcome. If it did, great. Either way, you just weren't supposed to do anything about it."

"I know," he said, angrily. "But that's not the problem. I did what you said, but Claire seemed impatient and her body was rigid. The whole thing felt mechanical. When I looked into her eyes, she looked away. Then she told me she was tired and just wanted me to hold her while she went to sleep."

"So she wasn't engaged."

"I was kind of relieved. But, Doc, your homework didn't do crap for me!"

I hadn't intentionally set Paul up for failure, but the unexpected result had revealed important information. Sometimes "mistakes" lead to answers.

"On the contrary, I think it did work!" I said. "I'll explain, but first let's go through your description slowly. Tell me what you felt when you began to *really* look at Claire?"

Paul gamely decided to play along. "I felt numb and even a little bored."

"What about when you first started exploring her body and focusing on what you appreciate?"

"I focused on my love for her, like you told me—and I did feel love."

"And when you looked into her eyes?"

"That's when I felt uneasy. I was really trying to see her . . . and she looked away. She looked away. I felt rejected—and exposed."

Paul's homework had uncovered Claire's reaction—and an answer. Eye-gazing is a great measure of one's comfort with intimacy and often reveals unexpected unease. I had asked Paul to put himself out there, to be emotionally naked, to be seen and to see her, to feel love during sex, and to share his eroticism with his wife. Claire had turned away, refused to see him. He was hurt.

Now I knew that it wasn't all Paul. Claire was part of the problem.

Paul wasn't conscious of this, but he had chosen a partner whose comfort level with intimacy was very similar to his. They had a homeostasis: When he reached out, she pulled away—probably to maintain their usual safe distance. Paul and Claire had high sex drives but a low tolerance for being emotionally close. In his attempt, however sudden, to make a connection, to experience love and tolerate vulnerability, Claire had tensed up and pulled away. Paul, and perhaps Claire, had what I call "love anxiety." Paul wanted to believe that he was in control of his world—at work, in bed, etc. Falling in love punctured his sense of control. We all have fears of love that lie dormant—often we're not even aware of them—until we *fall in love*. Then the question of our own lovability surfaces. Do we deserve the love we're receiving, experiencing? Because Paul felt anxious, which led to erectile dysfunction, he retreated to an environment that restored his sense of importance, power, and control: the massage parlor. However, the control was an illusion that Paul had purchased. The sex workers trolling the modern red light districts sold a counterfeit love—right next to the counterfeit purses, counterfeit perfumes, and counterfeit DVDs.

I wanted Paul to be able to experience and tolerate the real thing. "The real cost of going to prostitutes is that you're missing out on experiencing passion."

"But I feel passion for Claire *outside* the bedroom," he said, confused. "Just nothing when we actually have sex."

"The mind has a way of numbing itself to protect us from the fears we all experience."

"So, what do I do?" he asked.

Good question. I believed that Paul had to be okay with the power of love. He had to learn to share himself without fear of rejection, and to persevere in the face of it. "How about looking at this feeling as a celebration of the fact that you found someone you can really feel for. Instead of numbing out, embrace it. Convert it into passion."

"What if she doesn't return it?"

"That's not traumatic," I said flatly, meaning to desensitize the belief that not receiving approval right away is trauma.

"So how the hell am I going to get a hard-on again?" Paul laughed.

"It would help if Claire understood what you're trying to do here. You have to tell Claire what you want. Go home and repeat the same homework assignment. Maybe this time she'll be more receptive because it won't take her quite so much by surprise."

I never learned if Paul and Claire were more successful the second time. He had left the office saying he'd see me the following week, but he never showed up again. After waiting ten minutes during our next scheduled appointment, I called to see what had happened, but there was no answer and I had to leave a message. It's an awful and frustrating feeling for a therapist to just sit in the office, uninformed, when a client misses an appointment with no warning.

I took the subway home that night wondering if reassigning the same homework had been a mistake. Maybe I *had* set him up for failure. Maybe my intervention had been premature, rushed. I was afraid I might have opened him to a vulnerability that Paul, and likely Claire, wasn't ready to deal with. I had asked for something simple—for them to see the humanity in each other—but failed to take into account how difficult that is. However, I think if Paul was angry with me, he would have come back and given me an earful.

I tried calling Paul again before leaving the office. He didn't pick up. I thought we should have at least had a termination session to get closure on everything we had worked on. In the normal arc of therapy, there is the hesitant stage of getting to know each other, a bond that forms over time, and then an ending in recognition of all that took place. But Paul wasn't the type of client that needed to process the ending of our relationship, or even to say thank you or good-bye. I think he simply left when he was done. I felt the sting of having cared for him with no acknowledgment that our relationship was meaningful to him.

That evening, on the Q train, I watched the passengers packed in tightly, bodies touching, yet carefully and actively not acknowledging one another's presence. They read books and newspapers, listened to iPods, stared at the floor, or read advertisements on the wall, all carefully avoiding eye contact.

Everyone seeks intimacy, I thought. People want to be truly seen and known, yet we have so many fences in the way of letting one another in. Paul's emotional reaction to Claire's vacant eyes and unresponsive body showed that he truly desired intimacy. I hoped that our sessions had given him a few moments of the real connection he longed for, but as the train stopped and the rush-hour passengers spilled like waves onto the station platform, I felt swamped by the sad realization that in the end it was Paul who had become the "nonbeing."

CHARLES

Charles: "Tell me you want to fuck my best friend!"
Kelly: (tepidly) "I want to fuck your best friend."
Charles: "Tell me how you're going to do it!"
Kelly: "In the bathroom—while you're in the next room."

At my request, Charles and his fiancée, Kelly, a young couple who planned to marry soon, were role-playing the dialogue from their most recent sexual experience. Actually, Kelly did both parts while she perched on the couch arm nearest me, her eyes on fire. Charles, on the other hand, squirmed silently at the far end of the couch, clutching two throw pillows in his lap and barely looking at either Kelly or me.

Suddenly Kelly stopped and let out an angry moan. "I'm so sick of this. It's sick! This is all he wants to do: role-play me cheating on him. Every time! There is no variation except to replace his best friend with his boss, his brother . . . or even his dad. If this doesn't change, I am calling off the engagement!"

That brought Charles to attention.

"You know my sex drive is low, honey, and this is what turns me on. It's just play. I don't understand why it offends you. It's not like I want to pretend that I'm cheating on *you*. There's no threat here. It's just fantasy."

This assertion, that the world of fantasy and role-play is always harmless and should be indulged without scrutiny is an idea I encounter often from patients and sex therapists. I agree that role-playing can be a vital, creative part of a sexual encounter. An act of intimacy, admission to a privileged place. Charles defended this role-play as benign, but I wondered if it was rooted in something malignant.

Although I'd already had a few hours alone with Charles, Kelly dominated this session. She was volatile and reactive, often bursting into tears or anger. She dove relentlessly into what she wanted to say and left little room for my input. To her, emotions were facts. If she felt something, it must be true. No room for questioning the evidence or seeking rational alternatives.

Charles was a socially awkward, nerdy guy. He'd taken my sexual status exam during our second session, and it revealed that he didn't have a lot of intimate experience. He spent most of his time pursuing solitary hobbies like putting together elaborate model airplanes. However, Charles had his own successful engineering firm, and while the money allowed him to attract beautiful women, he confessed to being uncomfortable around them. "Mostly they choose me, not the other way around." What relationships Charles had had started with a woman showing aggressive interest in him.

In contrast to Charles, everything about Kelly was flashy and dramatic. Ebullient. Animated. Proud: of her career as a makeup artist in the television industry, her Italian heritage, of her Boston roots. She fit the type on which Charles had modeled his adolescent fantasies. Kelly had long, thick black hair and small, cat-shaped black eyes rimmed with a dark kohl eyeliner. Not a classic beauty, but provocative with her exaggerated swagger. With her tight-fitting clothes, full makeup, and designer handbag, she was the kind of girl who dresses sexy all the time. Even at the grocery store.

Kelly had made the first move with Charles, but it had taken almost a year to get to that point. The couple had started as friends, the kind who meshed easily, who could stay in and watch television in their old pajamas. One night she kissed him, and they took it from there. Kelly liked being hooked up with Charles because his introversion made her feel safe. And unlike the player types who usually hit on her, Charles openly adored Kelly. But now Charles needed the fantasy of Kelly having sex with other men for him to be potent, and their once contented relationship was in question, even though he took pains to assuage her anger. This was just fantasy. They didn't do it for real. They weren't swingers. They didn't patronize sex clubs. So what was the harm?

Kelly had joined our sessions about two months after I started seeing Charles. With typical gusto, she reported that while Charles was more emotionally reserved, anxious, and at times avoided sex, she was very sexual.

"At first, I thought it was fun. I'm sexually open and willing to try anything. But now this scenario is all he wants. I don't feel like the woman he loves," she said, tears forming in her eyes. "I feel like a blow-up doll. He's so sweet outside the bedroom. We're in sync. But during sex he disappears behind me—literally—avoiding eye contact. If I face him, he loses his erection."

As she spoke, I kept one eye on Charles, but he remained unresponsive, his expression opaque. Kelly had just said, in so many words, that she hurt badly. She seemed tired of repeating his very specific preference; his needs now made her feel as if she'd crossed the line between erotic play and Charles possibly acting out his psychological issues on her. But he remained still, didn't attempt to comfort her, and gave no clue about how he felt.

Because I practice sex therapy, my girlfriends like to ask me for advice. Some have inquired about role-playing. Usually, someone they're dating wants to try something "weird" in bed and they want to know if it's okay. I can't make any broad generalizations, because what's okay is different for everyone. I think the question to ask oneself is: How do I feel about this?

One girlfriend, faced with this question, decided to plow ahead with her boyfriend and be ambitiously experimental simply to discover where her boundaries lay. Her line turned out to be avoiding encounters that made her feel bad and that damaged her self-esteem—which is, of course, a very personal decision that's different for everyone. But it *is* a way to tell if a role or a game or a position will work for you. Examine your emotional reaction afterward. And don't just listen to your body, because even in negative circumstances you may feel turned on, or at the least your body will respond on its own. (A woman lubricating in a rape situation is her body protecting itself, not a sign that she secretly likes to be violated against her will.)

There's a blurry line between fantasy and reality. One girlfriend said her lover wanted to try spitting on her and choking her, but afterward she couldn't shake the sense that his desires had crept out of some very real and very dark place.

I believe sexual behavior has meaning. It talks to us. Sex is a blank canvas on which people paint their inner psychological worlds. The canvas can be covered with expressions of love and joy and celebration. Or it can become a giant landfill of unconscious garbage made of buried old traumas, neuroses, and fixations. The latter happens by a process of sublimation; unresolved emotions get rerouted sexually and show up as sexual desire. This happens often with men because they have limited social outlets and opportunities to deal with their emotions directly.

A good sign that this sexual chimera exists is that one gets stuck in a repetitive cycle, like Charles; the idea of cheating was the *only* way he could get off. He was fixated on this one narrow range of activity. Although this stuff seemed benign to him, as Kelly stated, these role-plays *felt bad.* In other words, the leaks from Charles's unconscious landfill had polluted the integrity of their sexual encounters, suffusing them with a general sense of ick. What was Charles coping with, or avoiding? Was this Charles's cry for help? I asked him to come in alone.

"Who cheated on you?" I asked before he could make himself comfortable.

He shot me a killer look, barely masking his surprise. I'd struck a nerve.

"What's the point of talking about something that makes me feel like shit?"

"So, something *did* happen. . . ."

"Yeah, but what's therapeutic about bringing up the past? It was a long time ago."

"Because it's not in the past," I explained. "Whatever happened, you're still living it." Despite Charles's resistance, I wasn't about to let this go, and I felt I had the right to ask. "Yeah, it's gonna feel bad," I said, sympathetically, "but let's confront it."

At first reluctantly, then with more and more energy, Charles told me the story of how he'd been engaged when he was twenty. She'd been the love of his life and he'd thought of her as "an angel."

"My feelings for her were so strong," Charles said, huskily. "I can't say that I even feel that way for Kelly. I was so excited to be marrying her. I've always been a monogamous guy. I always was—even as a teenager. I just wanted to start a family." Charles began to fidget, and his eyes darted around the room.

"But the day before our wedding I found out that she'd slept with my best friend. My best man. My brother caught them together. What I remember most was the moment he told me; it was the morning of the wedding and I was just getting out of bed, full of the purest happiness I have ever felt. And then my brother walked in and sat down on the bed and told me. I was devastated. I actually froze in place. I just lay there. My arms and legs were deadweights; I could barely breathe. I could hear the buzz of my family members moving about the house, and I could feel the warmth of the sun shining through the window, but I think my soul jumped out of my body in that moment. My brother told everyone for me, and nobody came into that room to check on me. They all left and the house fell silent. I continued to lie on the bed paralyzed. That was eight years ago."

His anguish was palpable, and my body absorbed the currents of his suffering as he spoke. My chest swelled, my eyes moistened involuntarily, and for a moment I had a loss of words. It felt like a powerful wave had come and knocked us both over, pulling us all the way under. We just sat for a moment, breathing, collecting ourselves. We both wanted to get away from the intensity, to keep talking. I could have escaped into some intellectual analysis, but Charles had been trapped for so long by this injury that no matter how much we wanted to avoid his pain, the dam had burst and he needed to endure and excise his agony.

"You were so in love. . . ."

"I adored her completely. I was completely open."

"And she just let you down."

"She *betrayed* me," he said, angrily. "Everything I believed was a *lie*. She didn't love me. I felt like a fool." Charles sobbed.

"She made you question if you were ever *really* loved. If *anything* was real."

"I lost everything in one day: my innocence, my dreams, my sense of reality—and most of all, the woman I loved."

That had been one of those life-changing moments, a psychological cataclysm, when the trauma of betrayal imprints on the psyche in a way that changes one's responses to the world forever. I imagined Charles's brain feverishly rewiring as he lay in bed, morbid and petrified. And the end result: a new association immediately and irrevocably attached to love. Fear. There's no trauma that affects one quite like betrayal. The aftermath is sort of a relationship PTSD, a fear that now defies all logic, infuses every thought, and generalizes to all women.

To survive, Charles rationalized an excuse to avoid the truth:

"I'm not good at approaching women, I get too jittery. I still don't really trust them. I decided they were all duplicitous."

"When did you begin to sexualize being cheated on?" I asked.

"For the first few months after that day, I stayed in my apartment," he explained. "My friends tried to help, but I didn't want to talk to anyone. I didn't know how to escape what I was feeling. I decided one day to calm myself down by masturbating. I was sick of all the tears and anger and found that I could imagine her cheating and it became arousing. I would think of her having sex with him and then get off on it. I know that sounds bizarre."

This was actually a clever psychological maneuver. I really respect the mind's subconscious ability to assert dominance over such humiliating emotions. Through fantasy, he was now able to control what had once been beyond his control. *Charles had eroticized his pain.* Literally, the shame transmutes immediately into a genital reaction, bypassing any conscious processing. It's sort of a mental victory, a fictitious triumph exulting him out of the pain and into pleasure. And every time he crowned himself with an orgasm, this relationship was reinforced in his brain, creating an inexorable bond between infidelity and erection.

He wasn't into role-playing for the fun of it. He was *trapped in the pain.*

I wondered how common this was, and then I remembered reading an account of a former call girl who wrote that one of her most common requests was to sexually reenact old traumas. Poor Charles, his erotic template had been tattooed. How was I going to remove this?

"Then you met Kelly," I prompted.

"Yeah, but I didn't even consider dating her. She was so beautiful and so popular, I determined there was no way she would be faithful to me. She was used to so much attention from guys, so I decided I would be her friend."

Charles and Kelly had nonetheless formed a romantic relationship, and now they were engaged. Unfortunately, Charles had been unable to leave his sexual past behind.

"Nothing else works for me, and the worst of it is that I can't even look at Kelly because then it becomes real," Charles lamented.

We made a plan to work through the trauma. I suggested we try to recondition his arousal trigger. I spoke with Kelly and got her to agree that part of Charles's treatment would be to avoid intercourse with her for a brief period. His homework involved exploring other thoughts, images, and fantasies that could possibly get him excited—even just a little bit—and begin to masturbate. I wanted to create new associations in his brain. Kelly was supportive, and Charles was able to successfully complete some exercises but ran into trouble on the next step, when I asked him to insert Kelly into these fantasies.

"What happened when you tried to masturbate to fantasies of Kelly?"

"Nothing. Numb. Can't even keep it up."

"Okay, something is blocking this. Are there any problems between the two of you right now?"

"Kelly and I aren't having sex, like you said. We're spending less time together. She's been going out a lot with her friends and I . . . I'm jealous."

I asked Charles to describe how his fears played out.

"I've been asking her questions about where she's been and who she is with."

"What do you imagine is happening?"

"I don't know. I'm getting paranoid."

"It's okay to have irrational thoughts and feelings. Let's take a look at them."

"I'm afraid she's talking to other guys, flirting, even cheating."

"Does that arouse you?"

"Actually, no."

"Great! This is progress." Charles was feeling his feelings instead of converting them into erotic fantasy. But my compliment fell flat. Therapy had started to draw out his fears, and with Kelly beginning to distance herself, Charles had begun to unravel. When he thought of Kelly out on the town, his biggest fear was that she would meet someone else. I thought I would work with Charles on how to talk himself through those tough moments when fear overwhelmed him. I suggested an internal dialogue: "We all experience insecurity, it's an uncomfortable feeling, I don't have to react, no big deal, this will pass, the reality is . . ."

Instead of focusing and calming, Charles looked like he wanted to smack me. His face went red, his brow furrowed, and he just stared me down as if to say, "I'm panicking and that's what you've got for me? A few trite phrases? A freaking Hallmark card for myself?"

He was right. Charles had tapped an emotional geyser that had been bubbling beneath the surface for the past eight years, and a few platitudes were not going to save him. What would come next, how he'd deal with the fury of this hot anxiety, was the real challenge.

Kelly requested an individual session with me. It had been some time since I had seen her, and I was wondering why she was pulling away from Charles and if she was still planning the wedding. She was upset with a change in Charles's behavior. He had begun to do something he had never done before, something she had never imagined he would do. Check out other women.

Oh, no! I thought. What is he doing now?

Kelly was attracted to Charles because he seemed to be the safe choice—the not-so-handsome, yet loyal guy who "should" feel lucky to be with her, and therefore worship and adore her unfailingly. This was exactly what she had gotten thus far, and it was her way of controlling her own anxieties about love. Now she felt insecure, the way she had when she used to date the good-looking guys and "players." She was incredibly resentful.

"Charles used to tell me all the time that I'm beautiful; I mean too much, even. Suddenly, he's stopped. He's less affectionate, too. And when we go out, I can tell that he's checking out other women." Kelly had worked up a powerful—and all too familiar—head of steam. "We'll be at a restaurant and he will literally be looking over my shoulder while I'm talking. I hate that I have to fight for his attention. Now all of a sudden, I'm checking out other women *before* he does, like I'm scanning for threats. And if I see him notice someone, I get mad. I mean, what the hell?"

"What does it mean to you if he finds other women attractive?" I asked.

"I never really thought about it. I've always assumed that I'm the hottest girl he's ever been with."

"So he shouldn't notice anyone else?"

"Yeah."

"Yeah, how dare he?" I said, illuminating her irrationality. But I knew how she felt. Kelly's reaction was similar to my own reactions to Rami's behavior, and as I challenged her, I was silently challenging myself.

On a recent summer afternoon in Florida, Rami and I had been at a party hosted by one of his friends. The huge house was jammed with good-looking people dancing to live Latin music. I passed through the kitchen and saw Rami in an animated conversation with a woman from Venezuela or Colombia—one of those countries where everyone is insistently sexy. I watched Rami speak to this strange beauty with a familiarity that made me uncomfortable. When he saw me, he called me over to introduce us. She was a friend of a friend, or something. I forget the story now, but I'm sure I thought about it intensely at the time. Rami acted excited about me, but when he offered to get her a drink, he sounded a little overeager for my taste. I stood there with a polite smile and then excused myself, went to another room, and sat down.

When Rami found me, he could tell I was upset. He wrapped me in his arms and sweet-talked me for a few moments. Then another woman walked by, another South American–looking bombshell, with long, flowing black hair and a curvy figure that was so sexy it felt inappropriate to even look at her. She was like pornography fully dressed. Rami lit up, stood, and called her name. I had no idea who she was.

"Oh my God, hi Rami," she chirped.

I walked away to talk with a girlfriend who had been watching.

"I couldn't be you," my girlfriend said. "I don't know how you do it."

That was all the validation I needed to get really pissed. Yeah, screw this, I thought. There was a constant stream of this—everywhere we went in public. Sometimes he would get phone calls from these women he claimed were "just acquaintances." He would say, so casually, "Oh, it's just Marcela (or Luz or Maria), nothing to worry about," as if I were a total paranoid psycho stalker for even asking.

The worst part was the excited look on his face when he answered the phone or saw them. He seemed so eager to impress. I felt robbed in those moments of what was special about me. I no longer existed as the dynamic and bright woman that I knew myself to be. Instead, I felt small and insignificant.

I started to lose my cool.

Soon thereafter, I got all rankled about Rami spending what I thought was too much time during the week with his new female attorney—lunches, dinners, drinks. I demanded to know why. "Don't be threatened," he said. "I made a new friend. Besides," he said, "she's unattractive."

A few days later he announced that we'd all be having dinner together. He thought it would help to introduce me to this "unattractive" woman. When she arrived, a big smile on her face, she was devastatingly gorgeous and I was ready to explode. But she was so gracious and earnestly friendly toward me that I held my tongue and stewed silently. After she left, I wanted to talk about it, but Rami just fell asleep.

I lay next to him, wide awake and steaming: How dare he fall asleep when I'm angry?

Impetuously, I got up. I went to the kitchen and collected a bucket of ice-cold water, stormed back into the bedroom, and tossed the water on Rami while he snored. He jumped out of bed and I bolted out of the room. He chased me around the house dripping wet, both of us screaming. Eventually, we started laughing, and thirty minutes later we were huddled together on the dry side of the bed.

We went many rounds of such folly, with the jealousy flowing from both sides. There'd be times when we were out on the town and he'd say, "You're looking at a guy! I know you are! You're smiling at him!" He'd get angry and wouldn't talk to me. Then he'd say, "Let's go, that's it!"

Then we'd get home and make love. This had become our normal.

After that incident with the lawyer, Rami and I had a talk and he admitted that he did try to make me jealous because it made him feel a little more secure—because *he* often felt jealous of me. When I calmed down, I started to realize that regardless of how Rami tried to manipulate me, it was really my own vanity that had spun out of control.

Kelly was in serious distress over Charles's behavior and I wanted to bypass the angry bluster. "What are you afraid of?" I asked her.

"I think he's losing interest in me."

"You mean that if he notices other attractive women then you're not attractive anymore?"

"Not attractive enough. I mean . . ."

"You like being special to Charles. In fact, you made sure to choose a guy you thought would cherish having you. Who would adore you."

I could see by Kelly's expression that I'd struck home. But she didn't want to dwell there. "All I know is that he's acting just like the other guys I've dated in the past," she said.

"Have you been cheated on before?"

"Maybe. Not that I know of. But I've been with guys who acted like they could, who threw their ability to get other women in my face."

This is a pretty corrosive dynamic. The constant threat of cheating may in fact be worse than the real thing. A subtle glance at another, an obvious gaze, smiling or getting excited about someone else, spending time talking to another woman, actually hitting on another woman in front of you. The weapon is in leading you to think that something *could* happen. Your worst fears are manipulated and then comes the inevitable self-doubt and questioning. Am I enough?

If you find yourself even asking this question, you're in a bad place. It's a trick question. You may not be asking yourself directly, "Hey, am I enough?" but the sentiment that you are not is present and causes tons of worry and uncertainty. I remember the moment when I figured out that I was beholden to that question.

It was a regular morning, right before work. I was going through the motions of my daily beauty routine. Everything was normal until I looked closely at my face in the mirror. Oh my God! I thought. I think I just discovered my first wrinkles. Twins, on my forehead, just above my left eye. I moved closer to the mirror to inspect the lines. Their length, their depth. I moved back. I turned my head from side to side to see them at every angle. I was horrified. Should I get Botox? Should I get bangs? Should I move out to the suburbs and retire? Okay, this was a full-on freak-out. I checked my face in every mirror, in every type of lighting. Are they still there? How about now? Sometimes the wrinkles would be gone and I was relieved, then they would show up again. I started to analyze my entire face for signs of aging. My left eye seemed to be drooping. My skin was discolored from sun damage. That's it, my life is over! (Or, more accurately, now I'll never be able hold Rami's attention.)

More and more, walking to the subway, headed for the office, I'd be in a bad mood before the workday even began. How did I get this way? How did a woman who used to walk through the world feeling pretty good about herself, so easily start to feel unlovable, unworthy, and unattractive? This is not me! I normally woke up happy; I had a spring in my step, even a little sway. Now I just stared in mirrors fixating on signs of aging as symbols of my lack of allure. How had I gotten so disconnected from myself?

We all like to bask in the glow of attention and affection. Someone's eyes sparkle when he looks at you, eager to know you, to listen to you, full of desire to touch your body. We want to believe that these responses are reserved only for us because of our uniquely enchanting qualities, because, like all humans, we yearn to be special.

Kelly now faced the fact that other women are also attractive, and yes, Charles might notice and could even leave her someday.

The reality of uncertainty and impermanence in relationships is a truth that lies latent within all of us, and we often rely on the illusion that our own specialness will create stability. Charles's new behavior forced Kelly to think about her relationship in a new way.

It goes without saying that our relationships with others are inextricably connected to our relationship with ourselves. Other people function like mirrors, reflecting back who we are. Mothers mirror their babies, therapists mirror their patients, and couples mirror each other. It is called—no surprise here—mirroring. The effect is to organize a patient's sense of self and reality. When, as a therapist, you reflect back the patient's strengths—positive mirroring—it has a beneficial impact. No wonder patients sometimes feel as though they are falling in love with their therapist.

Mirroring validates our existence. In a world of impersonal interactions, when someone wants to take a deeper look inside you, this is a powerful experience. The greatest compliment is to be truly seen by another. And when that person meets you with love and excitement, it feels powerfully validating. This is where authentic specialness lies—*in the connection,* not in the individual.

We instinctively want positive mirroring. It's an important part of our human dynamic as social beings and shouldn't be confused with indications of narcissism. Narcissism *can* develop if we have exaggerated need, and mirroring techniques can be used to manipulate: This is a brilliant skill used by many famous seducers. They go beyond superficial flattery by divining a person's essence and reflecting back its many layers in a positive way. ("Oh, I can see the sadness in you, it's so beautiful.")

The problem is that when a person becomes so dependent on mirroring as a source of information about him- or herself, all self-perspective is lost. At what point does the effect of mirroring take on so much power that it supercedes one's own sense of self? When you start wondering if you are enough.

Charles had stopped mirroring Kelly, and as a result, her sense of herself as special, beautiful, and loved had been challenged. I wanted to encourage her to hold on to herself in the absence of his attentions, and to believe that her worth shouldn't depend on his caprices.

Charles and Kelly started out with a special connection. But they lost all perspective as they got caught up in their drama. Now Kelly was fixated on why Charles would suddenly need to look at other women and was struggling with my attempt to redirect her toward herself.

One night at dinner with a group of girlfriends, at a trendy Lower East Side restaurant, we sat around a large table and I asked. "Do you guys get mad when the guy you're with checks out other girls?" A hot debate ensued, with lots of charges about who was insecure and who was not. A few said they didn't mind when their boyfriend's eyes wandered; it was natural and they weren't threatened. Some said they might participate by checking out the girls, too, or by preemptively pointing out a beautiful woman—as long as it didn't go on for too long. The others thought this behavior was poor etiquette at best, distasteful at worst.

One of my best friends there was generally unaffected by all of the cheating "horror" stories I would bring home from the office. She would always give me this look that said, "You poor pathetic soul, you don't get it." That evening she told us that she took comfort in a piece of advice her ex-boyfriend had told her, which was: "Men think about sex all day long. They imagine fucking everyone they see. Their secretary, the fat lady standing in line in front of them at the post office, their best friend's mother, the girl at the Starbucks counter with pink hair and a tattoo on her neck, their four-foot-tall accountant, and all the actresses on television."

How she took comfort in that I don't know.

"When I'm with my boyfriend at a romantic dinner, I don't want him imagining what our waitress looks like undressed," I said.

"The important thing is that he doesn't act on it," she said. "That's all that matters."

"Well, that doesn't exactly help my ego," I replied. "I want to be the most beautiful, desirable woman that my boyfriend has ever laid eyes on. I want him so captivated that he doesn't even notice the waitress with her gratuitous breasts right at his eye level saying, 'What can I get you this evening?'"

Given that my friends had been witness to some of the jealous drama between Rami and me, we all knew who the "insecure" one was—but I had a sense that this wasn't just about me. Yes, I threw a bucket of water on Rami, but what about the guy who intentionally incites this reaction in his girlfriend?

It was time for a solo session with Charles. I wanted to find out what his payoff was for making Kelly jealous. I wanted the answers for myself, too.

"Kelly always draws attention," Charles said. "Guys hit on her in front of me. And she loves it even while she knows I'm there, drooling over her, feeling lucky to be with her. I hate that feeling. And fuck that: Now I've turned the tables."

"But what message do you want to send exactly?"

"That other women are out there."

"And that makes you feel good?"

"Yes, quite frankly. I feel much better. She can fight for *my* attention a little. Let her think she has to compete." Charles bristled with puffed up pride.

"And how do you want this to make her feel?" I said, growing indignant.

"Lucky to have me. Appreciative of my love."

"How has she told you this makes her feel?"

"Angry."

"Doesn't sound like appreciation to me, Charles. Sounds like this is about what you want to feel. You keep her questioning her *own* worth instead of yours. You want to feel stable, in control, safe—but at her expense."

"It's not like I'm cheating. It's harmless."

"I think we should find a better way to handle your relationship fears. How do you feel when men pay lots of attention to Kelly?"

"Insignificant. I can't stop asking myself what these guys have to offer that I don't."

"Okay, Charles, I get it," I said. "You don't want to lose Kelly. But you don't have to resort to manipulation in order to feel better about yourself."

I suggested that the next time he felt like manipulating Kelly, he take a deep breath, check in with himself, and focus on his own value.

"I want you to try this: concentrate on *appreciating* that fear. That fear means that you love Kelly and don't want to lose her. That's a *good* thing. Try to focus on turning that fear into being grateful for your special bond. A connection that nobody else has with Kelly."

"I guess I've been destroying that connection?"

Charles wanted to take a shortcut. He had discovered that ego manipulation made him feel better and, further, that he could punish Kelly for *his* insecurity rather than work on dealing with the relationship anxieties that had been plaguing him for years. Now, by facing his apprehensions directly, I hoped Charles could truly effect change. He'd connected with the concept, and I sensed that he felt he could accomplish this goal. But a big issue that patients struggle with in psychotherapy is that emotional change does not occur because they talk about it in one or two sessions or because they've cried. There is no magical release and all the pain is gone forever. That happens through directly and constantly practicing and programming new ways of dealing with the emotions that come up again and again and again.

Charles reported slow progress during the next few sessions, then brought Kelly in. I thought we were going to discuss how to deal with jealousy issues, but Kelly had a different agenda in mind. "Charles," she said, abruptly, after we'd all settled, "I have to tell you something. When I went out the other night with my friend Justin, we ended up hooking up." Kelly looked at Charles with steely eyes. She didn't sound contrite. She sounded cold and punitive.

Charles looked like a deer in the headlights. "I can't believe this," he whispered. Charles turned his head away from both of us, his chest heaving.

"You've neglected me, Charles. I didn't think you were into me anymore."

"But I am. I . . ."

"Justin made me feel the way you used to make me feel. I needed that attention again."

"Kelly, I don't hear any remorse here," I interjected.

"You're right. I'm angry with him." She began to cry.

"You're trying to punish him right now."

"I want to break up," she said, with deafening finality, as Charles whimpered.

"Kelly," I said, raising my voice a notch, "I want you to stop. I don't want you to say anything else until we get your feelings in check."

"Forget it," she said. "I've had enough, all the weird role-playing and now ignoring me," she said in a full narcissistic rage.

"I knew it, I knew this would happen," Charles blurted, utterly defeated. "I knew she would eventually cheat on me."

Kelly stood, wiped her eyes, and walked out.

I had lost control of the session. Great, I thought, after all the work we'd done on the cheating fantasies, and now Charles would be re-traumatized. After Kelly walked out the door, he started to freeze up from the shock of Kelly's revelation just as he had that day of his wedding, lying on the bed. His eyes became hollow, his face dropped, and his became body catatonic.

"Charles, stay with me" I commanded. "Stay in your body. Stand up. Breathe. Stomp your feet. Feel, Charles. You're safe."

He clenched his fists and I could see his eyes reinhabited. He let out a deep growl, and I stood there with him as he went through several convulsions of emotion and, ultimately, fatigue.

Charles had elicited the very thing he feared most. He had re-created the original trauma. He cast Kelly in the role he needed despite her protestations. He idealized her, then asked her to act out the trauma in the bedroom, and then projected his fears on her by pretending he could be the philanderer, until he finally brought forth from her a rage that mirrored his own. A rage held captive in the deep corridors of his being by this erotic fantasy that was like a cork in a bottle. Charles had never completed his reaction to the original incident; his process had been stunted. He had experienced grief, but he never moved through the stages of grief; there was no anger or bargaining or acceptance—he simply tried to overcome the feeling by sexualizing his powerlessness over a woman's caprices.

I was disappointed that the cycle of reactivity between the two of them had led to infidelity. They really did love each other. They spiraled out of control over just the idea of a betrayal, and ultimately, Kelly acted out. I thought about all the ways we handle this crazy-making emotional jealousy. Charles, Kelly, Rami, myself. Nobody actually dealing with the fear—just passing it around like a hot potato. Many people live out their relationships in some balance between their need for love and their fear of it. But to clarify, it's not really fear of love. Nobody is really terrified of love. Love is great. It is more accurately a fear of losing love. Hence, we put an immense responsibility on others to make us feel secure. The reality is that nobody can guarantee emotional safety or fidelity, or make our insecurities go away.

Ultimately, getting a grip on our fears is an inside job.

Charles stayed on with me. He realized that he was ready to stop this cycle. "I set her up. I caused this. I need to work on these issues," he said. He fared well. He talked and felt his way through this time and was able to let go of the sexualization of the trauma. I get why this was hard. Jealousy, fear, and rage are a nasty triumvirate, and I can understand why he took the sexual bypass route.

Jealousy though, is ultimately about the stability of the self. Because self-worth fluxes and flows in harmony with relationships, we seek an equilibrium to maintain ourselves. Kelly cheated on Charles to reestablish her sense of self as desirable, an important part of her identity. The fact that she also wanted to punish him was a secondary gratification for her narcissistic wound.

As for me, working with Charles had helped me to face the very same concerns. I took a look at the slow deterioration of my self-worth and what I was doing about it. Like Kelly, I felt knocked off of my pedestal. However, instead of throwing buckets of ice water or moving to the suburbs, I decided to hold on to my own sense of value—no matter what. I could hold Rami accountable for his behavior, but how I felt about myself, that was all me. After all, I had told myself at the beginning of our relationship that I wanted to open my heart and be more vulnerable.

As for the "other women situation," I needed to realize that it's not fair to make comparisons. Instead of getting all wound up wondering how I rated, I decided to just relax and appreciate the gifts of others. I literally started to practice this. If I was out with Rami and some pretty-faced Russian or cute young Australian would walk over to say hello to her dear friend Rami, I would bridle myself, breathe slowly, and talk myself through it.

This was a very conscious turning point for me in dealing with the insecurities I had accrued. I didn't want to feel diminished; I wanted to embrace my own beauty, enjoy every minute of it, and take pride in my every step—regardless if he noticed.

As for the wrinkles? So what. This crisis was not about wrinkles. It wasn't about Marcella, Luz, or Maria. It was about healing the damage I'd done to myself. No wrinkle would steal my sparkle. I would look at myself in the mirror, not at the lines in my face. I'd look at the whole woman and remember who I was. I would hold on to my own sense of self-appreciation while in the presence of others that I admired.

This is what gives us the strength to deal with the vulnerabilities of love.

THE MEN'S GROUP: EUPHORIA

I got an email from a man I thought I would never hear from again. Steve was a moderately handsome guy and successful real estate developer with a nice sailboat. We'd had a brief affair a few years before I met Rami.

Steve's email was to the point: He hoped I remembered him; he said that he needed to ask me an important question, and not to worry if I was married or involved with someone. His intentions were platonic. "I live in San Francisco now, but I'm happy to travel to wherever you live because I need to talk in person."

That was it. No pleasantries, no updates on his life or questions about mine. I doubted this meeting would do anything more than entertain me over lunch, and honestly, I hadn't given a second thought to Steve since I'd seen him last.

At that time, we'd been on several dates when he brought me back to his place—a penthouse suite on the beach. Although tastefully furnished, the apartment seemed more like a sales model than a place someone lived in. I didn't see any pictures, mail, personal mementos, etc. He could have been a minimalist or just super-clean, but my intuition said otherwise. We lay on the bed for a while, kissing, but when he excused himself to use the bathroom, I jumped up and opened his closet. Totally empty! Not even a dirty sock. Oh my God! I realized that he didn't live there.

I confronted Steve and he confessed that he was married—with children—and that he had rented this penthouse apartment several years prior as a place to bring women. I was mortified. He explained that he was stuck in an unhappy marriage and that this was his only solution. But he didn't want to divorce his wife until he found someone he could fall in love with—and, he confessed, he had developed real feelings for me.

That hardly mattered. I could never trust anyone capable of such duplicity, so I walked out immediately. But Steve wasn't done. He texted and emailed me for weeks, saying he felt a special connection. He even offered, at great sacrifice to himself, to stop dating any other women. I would be his one and only. Except for his wife. What an honor! I could be like the favorite girl in a harem. Now all I had to do was oust his wife and I would become the queen.

I told him never to contact me again.

Now I had no reason to meet with him. But I was curious. I thought I might even learn something that I could use with my patients. I emailed that I lived in New York City and that he was welcome to fly in and meet me for a coffee. Steve wrote back that he could get away in a few days.

In the meantime, I didn't think about him at all. I was too

busy. In addition to individual sessions, I held a men's group once a week. We had five members, all of whom I also saw privately as well. Each member signed an oath of confidentiality so that they would be free to share deeply.

The group had no specific topic or prepared agenda. They could talk about whatever they wanted, and I never knew where it was going to go. There was also no structure, so anybody could talk, in any order, and it was very interesting to watch how they responded to this. I stripped them of any social roles; they were on an equal playing field.

There were often awkward silences, and this would draw out all kinds of social anxieties, especially the question of who was going to start, and who thought that what they had to say was worth hearing. Who would take a leadership role? Who would monopolize the group? And who would have a reaction to that? Or would any of them think they were a burden on the group? Did they feel like they deserved support? Could they receive it? Could they share and really tolerate that kind of public intimacy? Did they need to be the problem solver for everyone else? Did they try to take a leadership role or did they withdraw?

I thought it was fascinating to watch rivalries develop, and often someone would emerge as the alpha male, while the others accepted subordinate roles.

The members were Buddy, Oscar, John, Antoine, and Andrew.

Antoine, a French musician, was breathtakingly sexy and struggling to recover from a broken heart. He dressed like a young James Dean, and his personality mirrored that iconic rebel. An outsider, artistic, unconventional—all wounded and sentimental, with beautiful dark features and scruff.

Andrew preferred suits and power ties. He was often stiff, polished, and not good at small talk, as befitted a bank functionary or a square peg in a square hole. He'd been single for ten years, after deciding to leave his wife because he no longer loved her.

Buddy managed a post office branch. Thin, balding, self-important, and as pushy as his many opinions, he never met an argument he didn't like.

John loved women—to distraction. His preppy outfits belied a smooth-talking manner. Unfortunately, he didn't trust women enough to stay with one for any length of time.

Oscar was a guy's guy. He cheated on his wife compulsively and repudiated women in general. He was a building contractor who ran his own company and didn't hide his suspicions that I found him personally distasteful and didn't really care about him.

One night, Oscar unleashed a whirlwind of confusion about whether to remain with his wife, Nora, or to leave her for a young Ukranian woman. Shelly was his personal assistant, a recent immigrant he had hired off the books. She was also a single mom. They'd been sleeping together for almost a year, and he'd set her up in a secret apartment conveniently located near his downtown office.

After having been relentlessly indecisive in a month's worth of private sessions, Oscar decided to bring his concerns to the group. He hoped other input would help him to achieve some clarity. "I'm not sure if I'm really in love with Shelly," he explained. "Maybe it's just an obsession. But at least I feel *passion*. I feel nothing for my wife. I think this means it's over with my wife."

"What needs does Shelly meet for you?" John asked. He had

been in treatment with me the longest and often asked questions using clinical terminology.

"Needs? Everything I'm not getting from my wife," said Oscar. "Attention, affection, sex. God! My wife is so focused on the kids that she barely notices when I come home after work. Shelly will do anything sexually."

Oscar's provocative description of Shelly's sexual enthusiasm got the group's immediate attention. "What do you mean by *anything*?" asked John.

The answer was a thriller—and I hoped we wouldn't get sidetracked. Oscar explained that Shelly would make little videos of herself masturbating and give them to him at work. "I took one home and watched it while my wife was with the kids," he explained. "And she fuckin' caught me."

There was a collective groan in the room. "My wife threatened to divorce me, but I didn't just roll over. Before I walked out, I said if she wanted me back, she needed to fulfill my sexual fantasies."

"And she said?" I asked.

"She got angry," said Oscar.

And then it got worse. A few days after Oscar shared this story with the group, his wife, Nora, called me. "This is really hurtful," she said. "And instead of saying, 'Take care of yourself, I love you,' and something about the kids, he tells me I have to fulfill his sex fantasies and slams the door." Since then she'd watched the video—and a couple more she'd unearthed buried in a desk drawer. "The whore inserted . . . inanimate objects into her anus!" she said, freaking out. "I can't even tell you what else is in those movies, it's so disgusting."

Oscar eventually returned home, and Nora let him in, but she refused to let him sleep in their bedroom. Still, she seemed to want to work through their problems. Oscar, however, remained on the fence and didn't know which way to jump. Perhaps it seems crazy that Oscar was the one considering ending the marriage, but I suspected that a large part of the reason was his feelings of impotence in the relationship. Oscar had told me in session, though not in the group, that Nora was better educated and that her family had money. "I can't impress her with status or wealth," he complained. "That's intimidating."

I brought this idea to our next group session and said to Oscar, "Last time you said one of the turn-ons about Shelly is that she'll do anything sexually, and your demand to Nora was that in order for you to come back she had to fulfill your sexual fantasies. What do you think it means that it's so important to you that a woman will do anything for you?" I asked.

Buddy piped up before Oscar could answer. "Power. Total sexual control over someone." The other men nodded, knowingly.

"What are your thoughts on that?" I asked Oscar.

"What thoughts? That's it."

"You run your own company," said John. "Isn't that enough power?"

"It's not the same," said Oscar.

"As what? Acting it out sexually?" John countered.

"I think power changes people. It made me greedy for more power," Oscar admitted.

"That's true about power," said Buddy. "You get drunk on it and want more. You lose perspective."

"Was there a time in your life when you felt powerless?" John asked, glancing at me for approval. Oscar mulled it over. John, impatient, began to speak. "I think you . . ." I lifted my hand to silence him. John and Buddy, both confident men, usually angled to be the group leader and vied for my attention. Both behaved like model students, fashioning their questions after mine. They often got the terminology right, but that wasn't evidence of growth. John had strong competitive tendencies around other men, and Buddy was reactive to him. They were acting out their own issues, and if I wasn't careful, they would totally take over. I thought about calling them out, but Oscar seemed to be on the verge of something.

"Let Oscar think about this for a moment," I said.

John pouted. He didn't like being hushed.

Oscar finally blurted out an answer in a halting and tense whisper. "I was sexually abused for years by my older brother." He forced himself to keep eye contact with the group, none of whom were ready for this surprise. "And I couldn't tell my mother because she loved him more." No one was sure how to respond to this unexpected bombshell—including me, since this was news to me. An uneasy silence settled in the room.

"You guys are awfully quiet . . . " I finally said. The group often struggled with empathetic response, as most men do, but now that Oscar had risked being open, he needed their input. Oscar waited, looking embarrassed, and I felt the same. I was a little angry, too, that no one would speak up.

Buddy broke the silence. "I don't know what to say," he said, defensively.

"Wow, thanks for sharing that, man," said Antoine. I thought he had been silently brooding, but he had been listening.

"Yeah, that sucks, man," said John.

"Yes, thanks for sharing that. What inspired you to tell us this story right now?" I asked.

"I guess he controlled me sexually all those years," Oscar said. "Now I get intoxicated by being the one in control. For a while it seemed like I was in complete control with Shelly, but now I'm not because I'm totally hooked."

"Do you ever feel powerful around your wife?" Buddy wondered.

"No."

"I can relate to that," said Buddy, with a wry chuckle.

"My wife makes all the decisions around the house," Oscar explained. "I know it's because I'm never home, but I feel useless when I'm there. I'm just a paycheck to her. I feel like she doesn't appreciate anything."

I had heard this complaint from men so often that I wished I could pass it along to all women. Listen carefully: Feeling appreciated is very important to a man.

"So, it makes you angry when someone else controls you," said Antoine.

"Which makes sense given the history of sexual abuse," I said.

"I prefer a poor woman who appreciates what I give her and will do anything to please me," said Oscar.

"Which makes you feel powerful," said Buddy, who as far as I could tell authentically identified with Oscar.

"Yeah, and now I feel addicted to it, man."

Guys with power issues often create power imbalances, in both directions. They're likely to be attracted both to women who are, in their perception, of lower status, and to women of higher status. Shelly had, of course, been brilliant. She cleverly divined Oscar's power needs and capitalized on them. She would make herself into his sexual slave and allow him to feel all the power that he required. She would even humiliate herself. In return, he provided for her financially. But she was pressuring him to make their arrangement permanent. She wanted him to leave his wife and marry her. Oscar had made it clear to her that he would not divorce Nora, but Shelly continued pushing for that anyway. To up the pressure, she would tell him at work that later she and her girlfriends were going out to a nightclub to get drunk—while Oscar was at home with his family. Then, she'd text him to let him know how much fun she was having and that she missed him. Shelly never directly threatened Oscar, but she left him to imagine that the attractive woman who fulfilled his every fantasy was technically single and could be fulfilling the fantasies of any man she met.

The implied threat frightened Oscar. She was playing with his sense of control over her. He would feel euphoric each day that she had still chosen him over all potential options—even though they were an illusion she'd created. He would spend all evening preoccupied with what she might be doing. He had become obsessed.

It's actually pretty easy to make someone become obsessed with you. You simply feed the person's ego; then anyone becomes easy to manipulate. The key lies in one of the most basic principles in behavioral studies: reinforcement. There can be a predictable, scheduled reinforcement. For example, getting paid every Friday, or having sex each Valentine's Day. You know you're going to get it and that ensures compliance—to show up to work all week or to bring home a heart-shaped box of chocolates in February. But it also takes away some of the excitement.

Intermittent reinforcement is much more powerful. The schedule is indiscriminate. You have no way to guess when you'll get your reward. In this case, rats will push levers like little crack fiends, in hopes that one of the pushes will eventually yield a treat. For humans, intermittent reinforcement is like the slot machines in Vegas. Whether calculated or just street smart, Shelly had it all figured out. Give a little, then take it away. Leave Oscar confused, and when he got what he wanted again, he felt a rush. Yes, yes, yes! This is what Oscar interpreted as passion.

"Did you ever feel passion for your wife?" asked Buddy.

"Yes, for a long time. I loved her strong personality; now it's just taken over the relationship."

"You seem to feel a lot of anger toward your wife," I said. "I wonder if that taps into the anger you have toward your brother—and your mother for favoring him?"

"Are you saying I'm putting all that onto my wife?" Oscar asked.

"Maybe," I said. "Intense anger issues can rise to the surface and eclipse your sense of love. The love could still be there, just blocked from view. This happens often. People think the love is dead. In fact, the anger actually tells me that something is still alive."

"When something is over it's just over," Andrew cut in. "That's why I left my wife, and it was a good decision. I've been having fun ever since."

"So why are you in treatment then?" Oscar snapped." You've been single for ten years. What is *that* about?"

Andrew had a ready answer, no doubt by now second nature. "I just haven't met anyone with whom I feel that kind of connection," he said. "That chemistry. That magic . . ."

Andrew was the group's nominal outsider. He always set his

chair slightly away from the others. He only occasionally participated in friendly small talk before and after the sessions. He rarely said much when others reached out for help, and when he did speak, he would offer his opinions in a superior manner.

Andrew was also the most difficult to connect with in our individual sessions. He'd wait for me to make an interpretation and then decide if I was right or wrong. His manner was flat, with an undercurrent of anger, but otherwise he reported that he couldn't feel much emotionally. In fact, he drank to "heighten" his emotions, because "life feels like a barren wasteland without a good whiskey or a good woman." Andrew hated the banalities of everyday life and looked at me in the same way he did his whiskey and women—wanting me to give him something.

"I go out with women all the time, and when it's not fun anymore, I let them go. I just haven't met anyone compelling enough to make me stay," he told Oscar, in a tone that meant he didn't want to explore the topic further.

"Maybe you're the one who's not compelling," Oscar shot back.

I was about to intervene, but Antoine jumped in. "If you want to feel, you have to care about somebody, man. I know because my problem is that I care too much. I feel too much. I fall in love so hard, I can never get over a woman. I'm still in love with all of my past lovers." Andrew clenched his teeth and shook his head. "Andrew, in group you don't put in the effort to really get to know us," Antoine continued, "and I'm assuming you do the same with women. You have to get *engaged* in life, man. You have to open up to women, to see their beauty, to find the poetry. Every human being is a compelling creature—including you."

To my surprise, Andrew did not try to pick apart Antoine's analysis. "I thought I had the good life, a great career, a nice apartment," he said, shrugging. "But I never imagined I would feel so empty."

"I thought I loved women too much," Antoine said. "I fantasize about them all. I'm transfixed by their faces, spellbound by their lovely bodies, insistent for their touch. I get sick with love, I can't sleep when I'm alone, and I can't write without a muse. I can't function. When they leave, I want to die.

"But now I realize I simply didn't love myself enough," he concluded.

"I also want that euphoric feeling," Andrew said. "I know it exists. I've felt it before."

"Andrew wants to feel high." I said, to the group. "Is that love?"

This, in essence, is what each man seated in a semicircle in front of me wanted to figure out. They were all experiencing powerful feelings, but what were they exactly? Love? Obsession? Ego gratification? A cocktail of hormones? Was any of this going to be enough to sustain a lasting relationship?

"Antoine raises a point that is relevant to everyone here," I said. "What is each of you not providing for yourself?"

"I have an idea," said Antoine. "Can we do that group meditation exercise we did a couple sessions ago?"

No one objected. Each man closed his eyes, and I guided them through a visualization exercise on generating feelings of loving kindness toward themselves. This is an intervention I use often. It sounds kind of cheesy, but I don't care because it actually works. This time I saw tears in Oscar's and Andrew's eyes.

Steve flew in from San Francisco and met me on a Tuesday afternoon at a cafe in the West Village. I arrived a few minutes late, but he wasn't there, so I took a small table near the back, ordered a cappuccino, and browsed the *New York Times*.

Steve finally walked in wearing a wide smile and a few extra pounds, but otherwise he looked the same. He wasn't familiar with Manhattan and had gotten lost on the subway. He was quite excited, though, and slightly on edge. He didn't want coffee, or even small talk. "I'm going to get straight to the point," he said. "I'm still married and I recently told my wife about all of my affairs and how I was unhappy in a loveless marriage. She wants to stay together and try to create romance. I told her I'd give it ten months, until our next anniversary. If I don't fall in love with her again, I want a divorce.

"So, Brandy," he continued, taking a quick breath, "there's one thing I needed to find out for my own peace of mind before I put all of my emotional effort into my marriage. Let me start by saying that I have achieved everything I've ever dreamed of: great business success, world travel, affairs with hundreds of women. But I have never felt the kind of excitement that I felt with you. I've been thinking of you every day for years. Please don't lie to me, this is too important in my life. I need to know if you ever felt the same about me."

What? I couldn't even respond. But my silence made Steve nervous, so he continued. "I feel like I've done so much that everything has lost its sense of wonder. You are the most luminescent woman I have ever met. The world seems to light up when I am with you."

Instinctively, I slipped into my professional mode: "So, you want to feel alive again."

"Yes! That euphoria. It's magic. All the colors of the world seem brighter!"

Steve was ready to leave his wife to search for this euphoric feeling. But he was also scared that the feeling wouldn't last, and he wasn't sure if he wanted to throw away everything he had built for that high. So he wanted to know if I had ever felt the same for him, but all I could think of was: Is this what he thinks love is?

Is this what men—or all of us—search for? I understood. Euphoria was currently the topic in my group, and I guess I still clung to the notion with Rami. But I was also becoming disabused of it.

Euphoria is great. We should all enjoy it. But like my patients, and me, Steve wanted peak experience *all of the tim*e. This is obviously not a realistic relationship expectation. He seemed to be mistaking excitement for passion. He couldn't tolerate his own baseline state. And he had projected his fantasies about what love should be onto me. I pitied him. Steve was lost and confused, and stuck in the same place he had been when I'd last seen him years before. Besides being not at all interested in Steve, I had no desire to hang out with an emotional vampire who wanted to feed off of my energy.

I'm sure Steve could tell he hadn't won me over, so he launched into a story about how he had married young because she was the most beautiful girl he had ever seen. But he soon realized that she wasn't a match for him and he didn't enjoy her company. But it was too late because they began having children right away and he felt guilty about leaving her and them. In his mind, he was trapped. To compensate, he sought out other women and other pursuits, but he never learned how get what he wanted.

He said that in me he saw what he was looking for: a passion for life, an appreciation for the small things, the ability to find adventure in the everyday, a curious mind, and a desire to connect to people. The problem was that he was looking for that in me, and I wished he could understand that happiness comes from engagement in one's own life.

"Of course you feel very connected to me," I told him. "That's a skill I've developed. I get paid to do that. Maybe it's something you should learn, and try applying it to your wife instead of demanding that she dazzle you."

"You're trying to analyze my motivations, like I'm one of your patients," he said. "Listen, I just want to know if you felt the same or if I've built this up in my head over the years."

"I've never felt the same. I haven't thought of you at all," I said uncomfortably.

"Thank you for your honesty. You've helped me, thank you."

He walked out of the cafe, seemingly satisfied. I silently wished him good luck, but didn't hold out much hope. I never heard from him again.

MY THERAPISTS' NOTEBOOK:

What Men Want, Two Conversations with Michael

Guys tell me exactly what they want. They often plop down on my couch, cock their heads purposefully, and without hesitation, tell me straight out, "I want casual sex." "I want wild uninhibited sex." "I want passion." One gentleman put it this way: "I just like naked women," as if to say, "Listen, lady, you're way over-analyzing."

In any case, it seemed that my relentless interrogation of their simple comments often revealed complex truths.

Michael was a fun example. A single guy originally from Oklahoma, pithy and plucky, he loved to laugh at my fancy analyses and challenge me with a simple logic that was hard to defeat, especially in his cute Southern accent.

"I masturbate every day and I still need to have sex, is that a problem?" he asked, chuckling to himself and lightly provoking me for being so serious. Instead of analyzing his need to joke around, I decided to take him seriously.

Me: "How do you know that you *need* to have sex?"

Michael: (smiling) "What do you mean? I just know."

Me: "Well, what does it feel like?"

Michael: "I'm agitated and having thoughts about every woman who passes by."

Me: "Do you feel better when you masturbate?"

Michael: "No. Maybe I need to do it more, maybe I'm just a high-sex-drive kind of guy. How much is too much masturbating?"

Me: "I don't have a number for you, Michael, but if masturbating every day doesn't satisfy you, I don't think more is the answer. Maybe there's something else you want. I want to help you to be more conscious of your sexual motivations. What is it that you really want?"

Michael: "I swear, Doc, I don't know. When women walk by, all I'm thinking about is what they look like naked."

Me: "Okay, but you *feel* agitated. Let's be aware of what that could be. I think that sexual energy by itself feels great. It's an important source of vitality for people; our senses are heightened, we feel invigorated and alive. Yet you aren't enjoying that; you're frustrated. Why?"

Michael: "Because I haven't gotten any in four months."

Me: "But you get a physical release every day."

Michael: "Not with a real woman."

Me: "What do you crave about a real woman?"

Michael: "Touch, affection, someone to flirt with, talk to . . ."

Me: "Okay, so you're lonely?"

Michael: "Yeah. That's true. Just haven't actually admitted that to myself, I guess."

Me: "You're lonely. How is that to admit to yourself?"

Michael: "Sad."

Me: "What's sad about it?"

Michael: "I feel like a loser"

Me: "Because you're avoiding your own feelings, your desire to connect with a woman is manifesting itself as horniness. I think you're substituting one motivation for another."

As with many of my patients, it turned out that Michael didn't actually know what he wanted after all. Michael was clearly unaware of his basic loneliness, and instead, his body experienced the sensation of sexual excitation—a physical sublimation. With Michael, as with other men I've guided to be more aware of the actual nature of their desires, a whole host of emotional yearnings appeared to be weaved into what he thought he wanted.

I've seen this happen often in psychotherapy. There's some period of emotional intensity: a breakup, a relocation, the loss of a loved one. The patient is overwhelmed by emotion. One minute, he's filled with heartbreaking grief, and then, suddenly, he feels very lusty, and shortly thereafter, he has some blazing sex or falls desperately in love. The problem in therapy is that I know this isn't real, but the patient doesn't.

The mind has many interesting ways of trying to control emotional pain: numbing, dissociation, projection, etc. This particular mechanism is one of the sexier examples. It's sort of like taking the drug Ecstasy, and then, instead of feeling lost or scared, you feel like hugging everyone. You are not mollifying your feelings, you are actually morphing them. I try to teach patients how to be more conscious of their core motivations and emotions. A major buzzkill, I know.

Michael had some issues, as demonstrated by his urgency and agitation about getting sex. But he wouldn't find what he was looking for if he continued to believe in the chimeras of his own unconscious. Michael, as you've seen, had no conscious idea that he was lonely. And as you will read, there was yet another layer underneath the loneliness.

This example underscores the importance of sexual mindfulness. Sexual fantasy and even the physical experience of horniness often superimpose themselves on some other longing that represents something needed *outside* of sex. Why the sublimation? Why not just know what you want and go for it? Why the complex emotional labyrinth?

This next dialogue highlights why knowing what you want and just going for it isn't always so easy.

Michael: "I just want to have sex. I'm not interested in a relationship with a woman right now. I think going to prostitutes is just more pragmatic. I just pay, get what I want, no strings attached. I only wish I didn't have to pay and I could just have the sex. Why should I have to pay for it? Why does there have to be such a hang-up about it with women? If I'm horny, I should be able to just say to a woman that I am horny and ask if we could have sex. Why does there always have to be a relationship involved? Why do there always have to be emotions involved? Don't women get horny, too? Don't women just want to fuck?"

Me: "Have you tried asking one for that?"

Michael: "No, I don't want to bother with it. Finding women is hard, approaching them is hard. I have a hard time reading their signals. I would rather not bother with it all. It's easier just to call a prostitute."

Me: "Okay, sounds like what you have going for you is working out well, then."

Michael: "Except it is hard to find prostitutes who have the style I like, who are willing to do what I want."

Me: "What do you want?"

Michael: (pauses, seems uncomfortable, looks away, squirms around) "Ha ha ha. You're a little firecracker, aren't ya?"

Me: "Is it a certain sex act or some kind of interaction that you want?"

Michael: "Both. I want them to do things they don't want to do, that they have rules against."

Me: "Like what?"

Michael: (stalls) "Like kissing. Foreplay. You know, acting like a 'normal girl.'"

Me: "Like she wants to be there, too, like she needs it, too?"

(I had heard this desire before, several times.)

Michael: "Exactly. I want her to want it, too. Like she needs sex, too."

Me: "So, it's not just about the orgasm."

Michael: "Exactly."

Me: "You need touch, human contact, some affection. You're not just horny. . . ."

Michael: "I'm lonely, but I'm not looking for love, Doc."

Me: "I remember that you told me that a friend of yours suggested that you get a mail-order bride. I think this is a good idea for you."

Michael: "What? Why?"

Me: "It's pragmatic. You can bypass dealing with trying to find a woman or approaching one, which you say is hard."

Michael: "What will people think of me? It will look like I had to buy someone."

Me: "Well, another way of looking at it is that this is just your choice. It's an expedient and efficient option to deal with your dilemma. And, she will always be available, you won't have to deal with finding someone when you're horny, and, possibly, she will do whatever you want."

Michael: "She better do whatever I want. That would be nice, to have a beautiful woman always available to me. Hmmm . . . But, no. Then she'll always be there. What if I don't want to hang out with her? What if we don't have anything in common? She probably wouldn't speak English."

Me: "No English. That could work for you."

Michael: "You're really pissing me off, Doc. I want to find a woman I can be happy with. I do want to have a relationship!! Why aren't you telling me that I need to learn how to deal with my fear of women? You're advice is crazy. I'm about to walk out."

Me: "Crazy? I'm using your logic here. What makes you angry about that?"

Michael: "You're saying I have to buy someone! You're saying I can't get a woman on my own." (looking away)

Me: "No, I'm not. That's what you're saying."

Michael: (pauses, smiles) "Reverse psychology?"

Me: "Yes."

Michael: "I hate you."

Me: "C'mon. You're lovable. I know you can get a woman. Do you know that?"

Michael's wishes and fantasies revealed not only his anxiety about women, but a desire to *bypass* that anxiety. By carrying out the fantasy all the way, he could see that it was untenable. He revealed that behind all the bluster, he really *wanted* a relationship. The obstacle here was that Michael was actually socially awkward around women, afraid of them. He went for the paid interaction so that his ego was never tested. And when he tried to justify it to himself, it sounded pretty reasonable. Yes, men may just want to fuck, as he said, but clearly this was not his only motivation.

The reason that many of my patients don't know what they want is because they aren't paying full attention to what they're actually hungry for. They often have some mass of undifferentiated yearning for *something,* a sudden craving for a certain feeling, and they just act without thought. My goal is to teach them to pause when they have a sexual impulse and reflect on this question: What do I really want?

THE MEN'S GROUP: ANGER

"Women are bitches," said Will, a new member of the group. He stated it as fact, not hypothesis or a fleeting reaction. To Will this was hard-core reality. I looked around the room to see if someone would respond to Will's provocative statement. No one said a word. I wondered how many of the other guys believed this on some level. And honestly, their silence concerned me. This belief is not to be taken lightly; it motivates lots of relationship and sexual dysfunction.

I hoped that the silence was just a result of the group's social dynamic. Will had an aggressive alpha male personality, and the other guys didn't challenge him as much as they challenged one another. I finally addressed Will's assertion myself.

"That's a very one-dimensional statement about women, Will. I know how intelligent you are and that you are well aware that people are complex, so why are all women villains today?"

"Women have all the power and they know it," he said, staring at a point on the wall, as if in a trance. "They all manipulate, control, and seduce."

"So, what is it like for you when a woman tries to seduce you?"

"This one woman, she started telling me some sad story about her life. She acted like she wanted advice, but I have seen this damsel-in-distress routine before and I don't buy into it!"

"That's what you thought of her. How did you *feel* while she was talking?"

"Vulnerable. I don't want her to have that control.

Antoine spoke up. "What are you afraid of, man?

"Falling in love," Will replied, as if he were proud of having it all figured out.

In individual sessions with Will I'd learned that for him love was associated with humiliation and rejection based on his early experiences. He compensated by sexually degrading women and controlling them in an attempt to manage these emotions.

I was having a major problem with Will in individual sessions. I was bored. This had happened with other patients. Once past the opening tango of meeting, the novelty of a new story, of discovering a man's sexual secrets and excitements, of learning about the contradictions in his relationships, I can lose interest. I have been deep in the heart of my work with a patient, somewhere in the middle plodding through session after session toward building his self-esteem brick by brick—and suddenly felt as if I've already squeezed out all the tasty juice, leaving me just irritated with the man's struggle.

One day after a session with Will, I walked home and called my mom. "Psychotherapy is boring," I declared. "These men are freaking boring! Seriously, I had more fun waiting tables! Maybe I should do something else."

"Brandy!" she said, trying for a stern motherly tone, but laughing. My mom, I should pause to explain, is a beautiful Elizabeth Taylor look-alike, with black shiny hair, big blue eyes, white skin, and magical creature abilities to radiate love. She is a very spiritual woman who has given unyielding love to all—mentally ill folks, the poor, and me when I didn't deserve it. She has that luminosity that you often find in those who dedicate their lives to a spiritual practice; it's like some kind of energetic force field of radiating kindness. Just to give you an example, once there was a rapist on the loose in her neighborhood, who had been knocking on doors then raping the women who answered. When he knocked on my mom's door, she had no idea who he was. She invited him in and he ended up talking to her, praying, and crying. Then she took him to church. I always chuckle at the thought that he had no idea what he was in for when he knocked on that door.

So it's not surprising that my mother was quick to stand up for my patients.

"You need to approach them with compassion," she said. "Don't get discouraged. Be a light in the darkness."

"Yeah. I get that I'm supposed to be compassionate," I said, letting myself be soothed by her voice. "But I think something is wrong with me. Am I really supposed to feel compassion *all the time*?"

That sounded to me like some spiritual ideal. That can't be normal. Who feels compassion for everyone, all the time? I know I do my best therapy when I have compassion for my patients, but the truth is I don't always feel it.

However, I had learned how to go through the motions. I knew what to say and how to act, but trust me, patients can feel the difference. It's like mechanical sex: Two people can make all the expected moves, yet feel nothing. The truth is visceral.

This was a fundamental problem in human attachment, I thought; if they couldn't connect to me, the person they paid to tell the truth, then to whom could they connect? What kind of sex were these men having if they didn't have real abilities to experience a union with a woman?

I tried and tried to have compassion for Will, but it wasn't until he made his comment in group while expressing his irrational anger toward women that I finally felt it. It was one of those lightbulb moments: For so long Will had given me nothing to connect with. But when he honestly answered Antoine's question, I could feel the actual suffering behind his bluster. And I could relate to that.

At times, in sessions with men, I've felt like I was sitting with petrified wood, defectors from the human race, droids, their faces held rigidly in place as if stuffed by the taxidermist. Then I would leave my office, tired and defeated, wanting to stop trying so hard. But now I realized that it was this very group of patients that needed me the most. It was my job to draw them out, to help them to find their feelings, feel them, and talk to me about them, so I could care.

For any feelings to be present in the room, these guys were going to have to take the risk to let me see beneath the surface—and, I surmised, the same must be true in sex. The self must be present for sex to have passion. If what I was encountering here was some indication of their inability to form real attachments in all areas of their life, then I wanted to improve their ability to bond with me and the rest of the group. This would require an understanding that they mattered and that our therapeutic relationship was beyond a mere service, but a meaningful relationship, that they mattered to me and I mattered to them, that other people in their lives mattered, that sex mattered.

I decided then and there to teach them how to connect. Instead of getting bored and frustrated with them for not knowing how, I made it my job to draw them out, help them get real. I decided that the way to get there was to try and value everything about them, even that which I abhorred. They must have learned to shut down and abandon themselves, abandon me, for good reason. I would make a deliberate effort to take these men on a search, into their psyches and into their bodies, the murky depths of their chests, their bowels and guts, and draw them forward to give those places some warmth, some care, some compassion. I would look for the smallest sign of life, and direct my attention to it.

"I had a dream that I pushed my mother off a cliff," Antoine suddenly said. Whoa. This profound and primitive anger was so unlike Antoine. The group looked shocked, and so was I, but for a different reason. Only I knew that Antoine had been angry with me in our individual session earlier that week. I recalled that he'd walked around the office shaking his head in disappointment.

"What's that look?" I said.

"What look?"

"I don't know, Antoine. It's strange."

"I'm pissed off at you."

It's an important moment when a patient directs his anger toward me. There is nothing better than the real raw material being handed to you. It's an important opportunity for transformation—as long as I don't become reactive to it. I did have an automatic defensiveness that I wanted to keep in check, as this was an opportunity to meet that anger in a nurturing way so that I could create a shift in the way Antoine felt toward women in general.

"What happened?"

"You violated my trust. I don't think I can open up to you anymore."

"How did I violate your trust, Antoine?" I was truly confused.

"In group you mentioned that I have premature ejaculation. I didn't want them to know that. You violated my privacy."

I couldn't remember that happening. I never bring up a patient's personal clinical material in group unless he puts it out there for everyone himself.

Antoine did have severe premature ejaculation. The standard sex therapy exercise is for the guy to go home and masturbate until he's close to coming, then slow down, let it soften just a bit, then start again and repeat this process several times until he's trained his sexual response to slow down. This didn't work for Antoine. He could only last for about a minute, so even though he was only twenty-five, he started taking Viagra so that he could last longer. But he was terribly ashamed. We had realized he had a habit of eating, drinking, driving—and coming—without slowing down to enjoy these experiences. And we connected this tendency to his growing up insecure on the streets of Paris, never feeling sure if he would get what he needed to survive. And so he had learned to consume, rapidly and greedily, always fearing he wouldn't get enough.

"Actually, Antoine, I believe that *you* mentioned it a few weeks ago," I said. "Remember that day you talked in the group about how you do everything too fast?"

Antoine recalled but he remained resolute. "I don't think I can continue therapy with you. I'll look for someone else. I can't trust you."

"You don't trust *safety*, Antoine," I said. "You never had safety in your life. You were orphaned when you were little, and you don't know what it is to have a safe base. But you are safe with me."

"I don't feel safe now."

"You are safe. What you're feeling is exposed. And it's true. Because of our work I can see you. All of you. This is what intimacy feels like. It's not comfortable." Antoine squirmed a bit as my words sank in. "I can see how that would *feel* like I'm violating you, but think about it. And don't run away, Antoine. I want you to tolerate this. You are safe."

We had talked through the crisis then, and now he'd come to group with a disturbing dream. Where had this anger really come from?

"It was disturbing. I was enraged. I wanted to destroy her. I feel like shit about it now. Who wants to hurt their mom?"

"I can identify with that," said Buddy. "My mother told me that when I was a kid, I was angry all the time—but only at her. I think I once attacked her when I was six or seven."

"I'm not even talking to my mom" said Oscar. "She didn't believe me when I told her that my brother was abusing me. She gave him all of her affection and ignored me. She said I was just looking for attention, and that it disgusted her."

"Me, too," said Andrew "The only person I'm angry with is my mother. I know she's my mother, but she drives me crazy. Sometimes I can't see straight. She is so controlling and overbearing. I want to strangle her."

"I know. That's how I feel about my wife sometimes," said Oscar.

"Don't feel bad, Antoine," said John. "I have had fantasies about harming my mother, and sometimes I still do."

"What's behind that?" I asked John.

"She was super-critical and always compared me to my brothers," John explained. "I was never that great in school, but they each went to Ivy League schools. There was no way I could have gotten in. I never feel good about myself when I'm around her. I thought a mom is supposed to make you feel good about yourself."

The guys were sharing rapid-fire, not taking time to reflect on one another's individual stories. I could feel the hostility in the room and I thought about the power of motherhood. We all have major expectations about mothers. A mother is supposed to be nurturing and comforting, supporting, loving, attentive, protective. And when she isn't everything we need her to be, an anger swells like a tsunami in us, threatening to destroy everything in its path.

"As you guys can see, it is a pretty normal reaction to get angry when you don't get what you need from the people you love," I said, after everyone had said his piece. "The problem is that inevitably, they *are* going to let us down. Nobody can meet your needs perfectly or unconditionally. So what can you do with that truth?"

"Just don't talk to her anymore," said Andrew.

"Yeah, that's what I did," added Oscar.

"How has that helped your anger" Buddy asked.

"You don't know what she was like," Oscar said, bristling. "Besides, it's pointless. People don't change."

"I guess my mom is different," said Buddy. "I have a good relationship with her now. I just have to accept her for who she is and what her capacities are."

"Easy to say," said Oscar. "Why don't you try that with your wife, then?"

Time to intervene. "Okay, guys. There's lots of anger in the room right now; let's not throw it at each other. I think if we adjust our expectations then we won't get set up for disappointment. Women are not perfectly able to meet your needs, and that is no justification for cutting them off forever, beating them up, or cheating on them. How about a little compassion for the women in our lives and what their struggles might be?"

"How about asking for what you need from your wife or mother?" said John.

"That's always a good idea," I said.

"And when they won't do it?" said Oscar.

"Control them," Buddy said, laughing. "Tie them down and force them. They will love it."

"Come over here, babe. I'll give you some attention," John said jokingly.

"I'll kick your ass. How's that for some affection?" said Oscar.

"I say do it for yourself. You can meet some of your own needs," said Antoine.

"Yeah, I do enjoy making love to myself," said Oscar.

"Me, too. Three times a day," Buddy cackled, as the group broke into laughter.

Nothing like some good old-fashioned locker room humor to diffuse the anger.

That evening, making notes on the session, I marveled at how I'd been surrounded by a group of grown men whose childhoods had produced so much raw anger toward their mother. They had really worked themselves into a frenzy. I wondered about the nature of their anger.

Men don't necessarily walk around on a daily basis aware of childhood-rooted anger, I thought; they walk around feeling the very present frustration of needing a woman's love. What truly draws their ire is when they can't get what they want, because somewhere in the recesses of their being they don't truly trust a woman to provide. I've come to believe that this unfulfilled wish, for love, is at the core of their unconscious desires to kill, defile, punish, and destroy women. We see this portrayed symbolically all around us, and I believe it's an angry protest for authentic connection. As one guy said it to me, "I hate her because I love her."

It's just fascinating to me how much one's ability to love gets tied to this one individual, a mother. When a boy perceives his mother as uncaring, distant, or cruel, his entire view of women can become distorted, negative, and painful. Most of the men in my group had a broken relationship with their moms, and their own way of repudiating subsequent women in their lives. I don't believe they consciously wanted to be wary of females. When men use language like "whore" or "bitch" or "crazy" to describe a woman, I try to trace that sentiment to its origin. Interestingly,

I've found buried under the rancor a deep wish for romance. The problem is that when the women they desire spurn them, they experience shame and then project it toward her.

Moreover, I've also noticed that when women are promiscuous or treat sex with indifference, just a fuck, this word "slut" often gets thrown at them. Why would such hostility come from a gender and culture that supposedly lauds casual sex? Upon exploration, my clients reveal a worry that the sex, this intimate relation, is meaningless to her and, more importantly, that the man isn't special to her. Men may not always know it, but they want sex to matter, they want it to be special. However, some are too fearful to ever allow themselves to admit that.

Right before my next men's group, I met Oscar and his wife in a couples session. He wanted to explore the possibility of working through their issues. At times, she would communicate her feelings calmly and clearly, then suddenly burst into a fit of rage at him for stealing her life and her youth or for being a terrible father. I asked her to only look at me, not him, so I could soothe her while she spoke. Again she flung into a series of insults and attacks on his character, and I had to stop her and tell her that I couldn't allow this to happen in my session. While I completely understood her anger and knew it came from a deep place of hurt, I also felt badly for Oscar. I knew how contrite he was and how hard he was working toward change. He would earnestly open himself, and right in his moment of vulnerability, she would just knife him.

I was talking about the session with one of my girlfriends that night and said, "How did I get into the position of defending this guy? The cheater. I got into this wanting to help women." She laughed and said, "You are. More than you know."

When I next saw Oscar for an individual session, he thanked me for protecting him. He was touched. He said it was something his mother had failed to do when his brother abused him as a child. He expressed doubt in his marriage; he wasn't sure if he could deal with his wife's anger. I told him that she was angry but she decided not to leave him. He wronged her, yet she would still support him while he sought treatment, she would wait for him. Had he considered that this might be love?

Oscar decided to leave his wife and stay with Shelly. He told me this, making a bold declaration with an implicit caution that I shouldn't try to change his mind. I shrugged my shoulders, but honestly, I was disappointed. We had worked so hard on teasing out what love looked like, and what obsession looked like, and the differences. Instead he'd decided that his feelings for Shelly were not an obsession after all. She loved him. He was sure.

Two days later, Shelly left Oscar for another man. Now he was alone. That was also the last I saw of Oscar. He called and told me he was going to Spain and that was it. I was disheartened that our work hadn't been more successful, but this is what psychotherapy is really like; it's not always an end, it's often just part of the journey for some people. The process of change is slow, and I was learning to be patient. These guys would come in week after week, mulling over the same struggles and repeating the same patterns that didn't work for them. I watched as they got stuck in depression, anger, sadness, and anxiety, slowly plodding and laboring through the muck of it. However, I learned to view psychotherapy as an art, akin to sculpting; we carefully chisel away at an unformed mass until something exquisite begins to materialize, surprising and delighting us both.

I had a dream about Antoine. In it, I found a stone on the beach, worn smooth by the ocean. I wrote on the stone, "You are safe," and gave it to him to carry in his pocket.

I told him about my dream in session, and we discussed how he needed to hold on to a sense of safety. In fact, he would not be able to maintain a relationship with any woman unless he could learn to tolerate the unsettling feeling that goes along with really getting close. Whenever he wanted to pull away from me—like when he had imagined that I'd betrayed him—I told him that he had to get used to tolerating discomfort, which was necessary for his growth.

Antoine and I also talked about his belief in women as either idealized, poetic figures or evil temptresses who wanted to destroy his soul. "It's all fantasy," I said. "You have to get used to seeing women as they really are."

"How can I move past this?" he asked. "Give me a tool. What do I do? I'm tired of just fucking talking about it."

"Close your eyes." I said. "I want you to picture yourself as a child. Just go back and get an image of yourself as that lonely, angry kid. Try and see if you can really feel that again for a moment." I paused as he accessed the image. "This little guy is still a part of you, Antoine. I want you to talk to him now, as the wiser, older man that you are.

"Repeat this to yourself silently: 'I'm here for you.... I'm your safe base. . . . I will take care of you. . . . I'm always here. . . . I will love you. . . . You will have everything you need. . . . It's okay to slow down."

Then we sat quietly. Antoine's eyes remained closed. I wished I could hold him. Damn the psychology bylaws and ethics; sometimes they seem so inhuman.

I posed a question to the group. "What do you want from women?" I had been training them each individually how to identify their core emotional needs, and so they were learning how to answer this question in a new way.

"I want them to comfort me," said John. "I want them to make me feel good about myself."

"I want her to provide me with excitement because I can't stand being bored," said Andrew.

"I want all of it from women," said Buddy. "I want the status. I want to exploit them. I want to feel powerful. I want affection. And when I don't get it, I get pissed. I just move on to the next.

"The void is in me," Buddy concluded. "I can't help it."

"How can you fill that void instead of taking it from a woman?" I said.

"I don't know," said Will.

"Maybe make our own lives exciting?" said John.

"We can love ourselves, I guess," said Antoine. "Spirituality is working for me. I feel love from the creator."

"Yeah, gratitude. Appreciate myself," said John.

"How about giving love to others?" I asked.

"It's like the group, giving and receiving support from each other, like this," said Antoine. "Just letting go of judgment, no more competition, man. Instead, love for each other, for who they are. Compassion."

But I also knew that Antoine was slowly learning to do what he needed to most: to hold himself.

Speaking of lessons learned slowly, Rami had flown to New York to visit, and we went out for a romantic dinner. But that quickly fell apart when I realized that his old pattern had reasserted itself, when he started flirting with our waitress.

I'd had enough. I broke up with him and he flew to Morocco. Even though I was the one who had ended things, I took it hard. Weeks went by while I white-knuckled it through work, only to come home, lie on my pile of pillows I called a bed, and seek catatonia. Other times I'd play a sad song by Sarah McLachlan over and over, and sing along—loudly. None of my roommates ever complained until one afternoon, as I started the song for the hundredth time, they burst into my room, hairbrush microphones in hand, lip-synching the lyrics. They laughed and rolled around on the floor in make-believe agony. That got a smile out of me, but it didn't get me out of the house when they all took off for a party.

But one night my roommate Doreen had a new friend over, and while they were getting ready to go out, they came into my room and Doreen started offering my clothes to her friend. I jumped up, hair matted and sprouting from one side of my head, and began to scream, "Get out! Get the fuck out of my room!"

The poor friend was so scared, she left the apartment. Doreen said, "Brandy, that's it. You need to take a shower. Change your clothes. We're going out."

Soon I emerged from my room in an army-green tank top and a pink ballerina skirt.

"You're going to wear *that?*" Doreen said.

I nodded my head.

"Are you sure?" she asked politely.

"Yes." I wanted to look as crazy as I felt.

Doreen's friend wanted to go to a club in Soho, but I insisted on a lounge/dance club in the West Village. That night I met Khalid; a tall, dark, and handsome Egyptian. I approached him. He was fresh off the boat, having come to the U.S. a week earlier. He worked in his brother's pizza restaurant. He was twenty-five. He did not speak English. And so commenced a whirlwind, "nonverbal" relationship.

My friends, who adored Rami, but not my moods, could not accept this at first. I remember Doreen asking "What's his name again?"

"Khalid."

"What?"

"Khalid."

"Sure. I'm going to call him Pizza Boy.

I took Khalid all over New York. We were passionate, intense. I glowed, smiled all the time. Did I really know him? I thought I did. I thought I could "feel" us communicating, with our eyes, our touch.

Of course, my relationship with Khalid couldn't last, and after a couple of months, when Rami showed up at our front door, I was happy to see him.

CASEY

Casey was initially incredulous. When he called for an appointment, he asked, "What exactly is sex therapy? Is there . . . *sex* involved?" Is this guy kidding? I thought, but he really wanted to make sure that I wasn't "some sex service" and asked all about my academic credentials. When he arrived to the first session, I could see that he was quite self-conscious. Slouching deep into the couch, he reluctantly told me why he wanted help. "I prefer porn over sex with my girlfriend," he said. "What's wrong with me?" Casey's embarrassed expression all but begged me to help him find a way out of his predicament.

I asked a few preliminary questions and, as with all my new patients, explained the goals of therapy. I sensed Casey assessing my tone of voice, trying to determine if I'd be a good listener, someone with whom he could be honest and safe. When I urged him to expand on his attraction to porn, he insisted on telling me about his girlfriend instead.

"I'm madly in love with Amy," Casey said. "I'm definitely not here to complain about my relationship." Casey described her to me as a ladylike Upper East Side sophisticate with a regal air. Casey had been seduced by their innocent summer romance, nights spent strolling through Greenwich Village, flirting and laughing. "When we were together, I didn't worry about anything."

And yet only months after falling in love, Casey spent much of his free time alone, in front of his computer, staring at hardcore porn images of women who were—he confessed, when he finally stopped talking about Amy—unattractive to him. He particularly liked women who were in some way disheveled: hair tangled, makeup smeared, covered in sweat or semen. Quite a contrast to Amy, who Casey likened to a perfect porcelain doll.

"You probably think that's disgusting or bizarre," he said, "but it's how I get turned on." He added that he couldn't imagine doing any of what he saw on the screen to his girlfriend. As a result, Casey reported that he had lost interest in having sex with Amy. "She wants to have sex if I'm willing to just make love," he said. "But that's so routine and vanilla."

My involuntary and perhaps rude thought was that Casey *looked* kind of vanilla: a plain middle-American white guy in his mid-thirties wearing a blue button-down shirt and gray trousers. I couldn't imagine him having non-vanilla thoughts. Ironically, this made him even more interesting to me because I was excited at the opportunity to hear the fantasies of the kind of faceless man I passed on the street on my way to work each morning.

Casey's tastes bothered him deeply. "I am upstairs in my office masturbating to computerized images," he said, when I asked him to describe a typical situation, "while Amy, a *live woman* whom I love, is waiting downstairs. I think I'm this respectable man, and really, I'm just a pervert."

As Casey told me more about himself, I began to understand the source of his self-criticism. An Ivy League–educated intellectual, Casey was raised by a feminist mother. He took pride in himself as an evolved male who eschewed the traditional patriarchal gender roles. He valued social equality and felt uncomfortable "objectifying women." He possessed a sort of righteousness that bordered on moral perfectionism, and so he was disturbed by these sexual interests that conflicted with his consummately polite, politically correct self-image.

Casey's disdain for himself was palpable, and whatever swift judgments he might have feared from me could not equal his own negative self-assessment. However, I noticed that I wasn't inclined to judge him; in fact, my own fearful reactivity to the stories of my patients was waning. I had come to believe that all sexual behavior, no matter how dysfunctional, happens for reasons that can be explored and understood rather than immediately pathologized.

"You're really beating yourself up," I observed. "But let's consider this from the perspective that the reason you're looking at porn comes from a good place."

"What? I don't see how this could be *good*."

"Well, at the moment it looks like you've compartmentalized your sexuality. You're loving and emotional with Amy, but your erotic side is suppressed. Maybe your erotic side is also screaming for expression. Part of your vitality is fighting to save its life."

"But why am I looking at this crazy stuff? Is *this* my erotic nature?"

Casey had asked a good question. And I didn't know the answer. It's hard for me to know what someone's erotic nature is when it can get so muddled by viewing pornography. Because of the ubiquity of Internet porn, we can make the mistake of thinking that if men are looking at it and they like it, then this is what they want. We have to be careful.

Porn does not reveal some irredeemable truth about men.

Internet porn offers an endless variety of novel, bizarre, and hard-core images designed to provide an instant gratification not found in real life. Most people's bodies will respond to the images, and they have a powerful effect on the brain, each orgasm reinforced with a powerful mix of neurochemical rewards. An erection is a biologically conditioned response that can get attached to any kind of image one masturbates to, and Casey had conditioned his erections to the disheveled ladies of cyberspace.

However, none of it was teaching Casey anything about his erotic nature.

I explained to Casey that online porn is false eroticism. It's the product of corporate enterprise. A website's agenda is to compete for revenue by creating sexual scenarios. They take a variety of sexual acts and then they add a very narrow range of emotional themes designed to play with the viewer's psychology. The most common additive themes are demonstrations of power and anger. I have spoken to industry insiders, and they do intentionally pervert our common sadistic and masochistic impulses. While male viewers are complex beings, whose sexuality is not simply confined to two turn-ons, those particular themes deliberately appeal to a man's most base motivations. The porn merchants want to increase profit by showing exaggerated images of these underlying emotional conflicts because they are more likely to lead to compulsion. These porn execs are apparently reading Freud.

I know that the pro-pornography folks argue that it's supposed to be selling fantasies for harmless adult titillation or inspiration, but the effect on some of my clients is alienation from themselves and the real people they're sleeping with. My girlfriends used to joke about guys who overindulged in porn. Usually we could immediately tell where guys we dated got their attitudes in bed. If we dated someone who seemed bent on acting out fantasy scenarios instead of showing any real interest in connecting with us, we'd say, "I went out with a porn guy." These were the guys who wanted to play the schoolgirl fantasy the first or second time they ever slept with one of us. I was glad that my man had grown up on *Playboy* instead of the Internet. There was a big difference.

Another friend of mine went on a few dates with a young medical resident, and after they slept together she told me that the experience was at first very sweet and sensual and she thought they were expressing their mutual like for each other until out of nowhere he said, "Tell me you're a sexy bitch!"

"I was so startled that I froze," she said. The outburst was so arbitrary and incongruent with the moment, and with the feelings she had begun to develop for her date, that she never went out with him again—even though he kept calling.

I wondered about this disconnect between men and women in the meaning of sex. Is it an act of intimacy, a game, or both? When it came to the reality of the pervasiveness of porn, I, of course, preferred not to think about it. I wanted to live in my own reality, my own construction of what various sex acts meant to me. I didn't consider that my partner might have very different ideas. I had a kind of "not in my backyard" mentality. At least I knew that Rami wasn't looking at porn while I waited for him in the bedroom. But I wondered if he used it when I wasn't around. We were, after all, in a long-distance relationship.

Being my impulsive self, I decided to call him. "Rami," I asked, "when you're not with me, do you look at porn?"

"Yes," he said, without hesitation.

No! I thought. I had a flash flood of irrational thoughts. A betrayal! How dare he have a secret world that I don't know about! How dare he not let me know his every thought and desire! My sense of reality was punctured for a minute. Then I pulled it together.

"What kind of porn?" I asked, feigning being totally cool and unaffected.

"I'll turn on Showtime a couple times a week and watch an adult movie."

That soft-core stuff was fine. "What about on the Internet?"

"Not on the computer. I don't understand how to use it."

"Do you masturbate when you watch?"

"Sometimes," he said, matter-of-factly.

The next time I spent the weekend at his place in Florida, I was struck by a moment of paranoia. I went into Rami's bedroom and started snooping around. In a drawer I found a stack of what looked like home-burned DVDs with half-naked young women on the labels. I freaked out. Discs in hand, I confronted him. "Those were given to me by Yousif," he explained, when I dropped them on the table in front of him. Yousif was one of

Rami's married friends. I'd always thought he was sleazy, and he could drive me crazy. "Yousif is a pervert," Rami said. "He looks at porn all day long in his office. He made copies and gave them to me. I swear to God, I've never even watched them."

"Then why didn't you throw them away?"

Rami didn't answer, but he got rid of them immediately.

I could have analyzed forever why he'd kept the discs, but I settled on acceptance for my own peace of mind. I tried to remember not to fall into the trap of thinking that I was somehow deficient because he enjoyed what he saw.

I thought about this other twenty-four-year-old male patient who, like Casey, came to see me because he was concerned that watching too much Internet porn lowered his interest in his girlfriend. He said that he was so in love with her yet sexually he could only think of what he had seen online. He said he felt "polluted" and wanted to meet her from a "better place." That seemed a mature statement for someone so young. When I asked him to describe his sex life *before* he first watched porn, he said, "I've never *not* had Internet porn as part of my life."

Wow. I marveled at how the omnipresent Internet must have shaped his desires; the two seemed inextricably linked, and this young man wanted to untether his sexuality. This young man wanted to become more conscious about his sexuality, and I wondered if it were possible for him and Casey to liberate their yearnings from what they'd been taught to like, or if they should just accept what turns them on and share it with their partners.

I asked Casey if he'd ever shared the side of himself that liked porn with Amy.

"I can tell she wouldn't be into that."

"So you tried?"

"She is more romantic, into making love."

"So you didn't."

Casey wanted to shake off the question. "I tried a little. I suggested a few things," he said. "But look: I really respect and admire her. I wouldn't feel comfortable doing any of the stuff with Amy that I see online. I don't want her to know about all the crazy shit I look at, okay? And there's just some stuff I wouldn't do with her. I just respect her too much."

"Of course you don't want to act out *most* of that stuff with her, but the important point is not the content of the images you look at; rather it's that eroticism seems to be missing from the relationship. *Not* sharing your erotic side creates at least part of the disconnection here."

"Don't you see? I love Amy and I want to be turned on by making love to her," he said. "But I'm being honest with you here: I get bored with that."

"So you think making love is boring, but you want me to help you get turned on by it? I think you're bored because you're not being erotic enough."

"I don't want to offend her."

"Why would that be bad?"

Casey gave me sharp look as if to ask, "Where is this going?" We had begun to misunderstand each other.

I was trying to get Casey to realize that his fear of Amy's reaction was a part of the problem here. He was so concerned about what she'd think that his erotic desires were suppressed and then sublimated, emerging elsewhere with pornography.

But I would never get Casey to put together the two disparate pieces of his sexuality unless I got rid of his shame. I wanted him to let go of the self-judgment so we could do some real exploration. So I asked Casey to consider his idea of "crazy shit" for a moment. What did it really mean? "I've listened to many sexual fantasies and learned that what turns people on is usually less than politically correct," I explained. "The weird, the disgusting, the exploitive—it often surprises and confuses us. But what seems to bother you *most* is hoping that your erotic desires are not really you—and you worry that they are."

In order to become more sexually conscious, he first needed to accept that humans are simply wired to respond to sexual imagery of all kinds. So he got an erection—nothing to freak out about.

Casey was caught up in the content of porn, but it wasn't the content that mattered here; it was his personal relationship with it. Porn can serve various psychological functions. Those who use porn in lieu of actual sexual engagement effectively bypass their intimacy anxiety. Porn feels safer. There's no rejection. You can have sex with any woman you want. She is always ready and willing to do whatever you wish. There's no emotional attachment, no judgment, and no pressure to perform. And best of all, she's always excited to be with you.

Casey thought his affection for porn had caused the problem, but it went deeper. Casey had to come to terms with the fact that he was indeed an erotic being. We just had to figure out what that meant. Otherwise he'd remain caught in a cycle of repression and acting out. I didn't want to push him to share with Amy at this point; I only wanted him to see that the lack of communication was part of the reason for his fractured sexual identity. Casey still had lots of work to do on himself. I wanted to get beyond the superficial cultural conditioning and his psychology to get to the essence of who he was sexually. I wanted to see if he could find his own creativity, and this would involve some conscious exploring rather than passively responding to what was most easily available.

We decided to explore his sexual development. When Casey's parents, both Woodstock generation hippies, talked to him about sex, they emphasized the need to respect women and to view the sexual act as sacred. "I agreed with that," he said. "I still want that ideal. But as a teenager, I wasn't having much sex, so bootleg movies from my friends were the next best thing. I've been looking at porn for so long and honestly just considered it normal male behavior," he said.

"So you learned to go straight to porn for an erotic release. What has that really taught you about yourself?"

Casey laughed. "That I get turned on by doing things my mom said not to do?"

Of course, the subversive act in opposition to one's ideals can be inherently sexy. But where had that "disheveled" look Casey liked come from? Certainly not from his mother or girlfriend.

"Seriously, Casey, what have you learned about yourself?"

"If I really think about it . . . what I notice . . . hmmm . . . I guess I get turned on by aggression, domination, the lack of feeling involved. It's hard to admit that," Casey continued, "because it goes against everything I've wanted to believe."

Casey was perplexed. "But I don't have any weird power issues with my parents, I swear. I don't feel powerless in my life. I don't feel insecure about Amy. I just like it."

Frankly, the idea of men furtively excited by viewing females in powerless positions was uncomfortable for me to hear, especially from the most socially conscious of my male clients. Perhaps deep analysis was unnecessary. Maybe it was simple: Power feels good. And porn offered him/men a way to dominate and enjoy it. "Possibly at the expense of the woman," I said.

"'At the expense of a woman.' Wow, it sounds selfish when put that way," Casey said. "But men get a lot of reinforcement for being in control of a woman. It's status."

This seemed to me a cheap way to feel good. From the time I encountered a stash of girlie magazines in a "fort" shared by neighborhood boys, I was curious about what men looked at and why they shared it with one another. I thought it could be a form of storytelling about masculinity, with messages that got passed down through generations. If so, maybe I could turn around this cultural trope about domination, if only for one man. In his desperation to come to terms with himself, Casey seemed open enough, and I was grateful that he was willing to explore the topic. Typically, I had found guys rather defensive about porn, ready to minimize its deleterious effects. It was as if I was poking at the sacred cow, some sacred right, that women should just accept as nonthreatening male normality and never question. "Men give each other messages that shape what they think is sexy," I said. "But where in this is the real you?"

"Never thought about it. How do I find myself?"

"What if you start with considering other sources of eroticism other than online porn?"

"Like?"

"Erotic literature, erotic poetry, Tantra, your own imagination . . . ?"

"Maybe I could even get Amy on board with *that,*" he said. "It would seem more like making love . . ."

Now we had circled back. What Casey wanted was to have a sexual relationship with Amy that included acts he also found erotic. Fine. Eroticism isn't bad. The problem was his separation of love and eroticism.

I wasn't sure where his exploration might lead. I didn't have any real plan for him yet. I just believed there had to be a way for Casey and Amy to be erotic together, something he could integrate into his identity, his ideals, his love for Amy. I couldn't speak for Amy since I only had Casey's point of view, but he was obviously inhibited by her. He didn't feel the emotional safety to explore himself in her presence. The fact that porn was successful in drawing him out, and led to temporary satisfaction, only created confusion about what he wanted. I hoped we could stop this cycle and construct a bridge over the partition of his identity.

I had my own ideas about what constituted erotic sex and had to be thoughtful and careful about imposing them on Casey. I liked the idea of celebrating the act, celebrating each other's body. I resented the most common theme in porn that took the penis and semen and turned them into weapons of destruction, when, after all, their real function is to create life.

I generally define "the erotic" as a carnal, animal, physical, or pleasure-based experience. It's a pervasive earthy, elemental sensuality. It's not actually separate from love, as Casey seemed to think, but it *is* separate from the soft-focus and lace concept of love, which Casey believed Amy was more attached to.

When thinking about our erotic nature, it's important to remember the influence of the cultural context. It's too reductive to simply look around at modern mores and make generalizations. In my studies on historical and cross-cultural trends in sexual expression, I discovered a huge range. I once thought that power play was a universal turn-on, until I discovered popular traditions, including Taoism, Tantra, and pre–major religion European culture, that were very sex-affirmative for *both* men and women (then this changed in each of these cultures). But it's important to note that there was a significant period in human history when people didn't seem to need themes of dominance to get turned on. In ancient China, during the popularity of Taoist thought, there's almost no evidence of sadomasochistic behavior, and male and female sexual anatomy was not referred to pejoratively as it is now. Instead of "prick" or "cunt," they used words like "jade stem" and "jade vase." Women were regarded as highly sexual and their orgasms were thought to bring health and vitality to both sexes, so men were often trained in how to keep women satisfied.

Even ancient art reflected these ideas. Looking through a book on the topic, I compared the European prehistoric art images of women to modern porn. There appeared to be no suggestion of obscenity or even the concept of obscenity in the ancient material. The nude images of breasts and body were fertility symbols. Sex simply celebrated life. Meanings attached to sex were about creation, abundance, potency, and life force.

I like these ancient perspectives. I actually find them very erotic; the pagans out in the fields having sex, hoping to help the fertility of the soil, is a sexy idea. I also discovered that women have historically been perceived as very sexual, even more so than men. I like to imagine how this cultural context impacted women's libidos. In fact, the notion that women are less sexual than men is only a few hundred years old. In European history, women were considered very sexual until feudalism fell and capitalism emerged. Soon sexually aggressive women could be burned as witches, and Western women were henceforth brought up to be passive and to mirror their husbands' desires.

So my point is that cultural context is very important in understanding men's sexual behavior, because it in some part expresses what's in the social environment. Currently, our psyches are strongly inculcated with dominance, competition, and power.

When Casey arrived for his next session, I could immediately tell that something had happened. He started talking even before we reached the office, in a way that was markedly different from the controlled, cerebral, self-recriminating man I'd come to know. It was as if some spigot had been opened, as if he'd pressed the "screw it" button and decided to be free, to shed the dead skin of self-consciousness and reveal an animated, vibrant spirit.

"I figured it out," he said brightly. Casey's voice was sure, his eyes wide, his posture confident. "I was walking through Washington Square this morning and I saw a woman. I noticed her body like I would notice any attractive woman walking by. But I turned and followed her. It was impulsive; I never do that. But I started following her, and I couldn't take my eyes off the shape of her ass as she walked ahead of me."

"How did you feel?"

"Hot inside. I felt like an animal on the hunt, and I just wanted to pounce on her and fuck her." Suddenly, the Casey I knew appeared. "Is this offensive?

"I appreciate your honesty," I said. "You're getting real here, that's a step," Impacted by his passion sparking through the room like an electrical current, I even felt a bit aroused.

"I just wanted to let myself feel like I did without censoring myself."

"What did you figure out?"

"I felt like I could have devoured that woman. I wanted to be forceful, to penetrate. I could have pushed her up against a tree and bit right into her flesh. I wasn't angry—just primal, I guess. I felt kind of guilty, but I'm tired of that soft and slow routine. I'm hungry. I want to fuck!" he declared in a low growl.

I was a bit unnerved by his intensity. I adjusted my position in my chair, bridling myself, upright and leaning to the side, suddenly aware of my own curves as I caught his eyes drifting down the side of my body when I twisted my waist. Later, I wondered if I was unconsciously displaying myself—if somewhere deep in my own primal nature I was responding to him.

"Guilty? About?" I asked, refocusing the both of us.

"I thought the whole point of this was that you wanted me to find my softer side so I would fit better with Amy."

"No. I wanted you to find the real you. Aggressive impulses aren't bad, Casey. They reflect your passion."

"I felt like: This is what I want, this is who I am!"

"Let's celebrate the humanity in that urge. This is what vitality is all about. But the next question is: Can you direct this toward Amy?"

"Normally, no. But . . . I think I'm ready to try."

Although Casey had originally been seduced by Amy's romanticism, he'd grown weary of what he perceived as her limits on lovemaking, which was only that: *lovemaking.* Casey wanted to fuck. He remembered how he used to fuck women and he wanted more. He had a deep desire to plunder flesh, to penetrate vigorously, but he was blocked by Amy's gentility and his fear of sundering it. But today he'd expressed healthy aggression, different from porn aggression, that poisonous rage mixed with hatred, sadism, and subversion. Casey felt positive about passion inflamed by savage corporeal magnetism and he was willing to own it.

Casey went out of town for a couple of weeks, and the next time he made an appointment he called to see if I'd let him bring his beloved lady, Amy. Of course, I was curious.

When they arrived, I could see why he was so taken with her. Amy had a powerful presence. She moved her body with the graceful deliberation of a ballet dancer, shoulders pulled back proudly, head held high. The effect showcased the delicate curves of her lithe figure.

I was caught off guard when I walked out into the waiting room and discovered that she didn't have wings, or a halo, or a long, flowy, diaphanous dress. Instead, Amy wore a high-fashion ensemble, expensive and artistic—but not necessarily flattering. She made the kind of style choices that draw more attention from women than men. She was also so meticulously coiffed and manicured that she seemed oddly disconnected from any sense of raw sensuality. Being around Amy was like being in one of those perfectly clean, almost staged houses where you admire the aesthetic, but don't feel comfortable sitting down.

I was smiling and almost ingratiating in my warmth as I welcomed her to my office, yet she was cursory in greeting me, which felt disappointing; I was ready to soak in her much reputed charm. Casey and Amy didn't look so amorous as they entered my office and sat down. I couldn't imagine the mentioned walks in the West Village as they sat on opposite ends of the couch, his body language defeated and hers tense and closed off. Both avoided eye contact and only addressed me. Her first order of business was to let me know how "screwed up" my patient is, as if she was telling on him or reproaching me, I couldn't quite tell. Her speech was pressured and her tone castigating, her grace fading as her anxiety rose.

"Something has changed in him," she said, disparagingly. "He's so sex-crazed, constantly suggesting new positions, new places, bondage, etc. I can understand that he wants to spice it up, but to be honest, it seems like all he cares about is sex. Is this why he's been seeing you? Is this what you're telling him to do?"

Instead of answering, I asked, "How do you feel about that?"

Amy sloughed off my question in return. "And worse, he asked me to look at porn with him." No wonder Casey looked so glum.

"I feel betrayed," Amy continued. "What? I'm not enough anymore?" She posed the question to me, but meant it for Casey. He looked away.

"Sounds like you're not feeling loved by Casey right now."

"There's nothing loving about it. I feel like I'm being used."

"Is it possible that he wants to spice up the sex *because* he loves you?"

"What? This is the way he shows love?" she asked sarcastically.

"Outside of his recent sexual behavior, do you have evidence or reason to believe that Casey doesn't love you?"

"None. That's why this is confusing for me."

"What are you afraid this means?"

"That he's falling *out* of love with me. That he doesn't care anymore. I think he just wants to use me to get off."

"That's a strong assumption."

Amy glared at me.

"Could it be that Casey asking you to share his erotic side is an act of intimacy?"

Casey sulked in a shame-induced slump as Amy's anger stirred up his guilt and blocked his quest for authenticity that we'd long worked on. I wished he would help me by speaking up, but he cowered in the face of her frustration.

"Have you guys had a discussion about these changes in your sex life?"

"We don't talk about our sex life," said Amy.

"Why not?"

"If we're in love, then it will naturally be good."

I held my tongue and let her declaration hang in the air. "That is a dangerous myth, Amy," I finally said. "Sex is *not always* good, even when two people are deeply in love." They both looked at me as if they'd never heard anything that preposterous before—or at least had not believed it. "If there's no communication, you leave yourselves open to all kinds of misinterpretations. Casey, you imposed your new ideas on Amy *without* checking in with her. She has no idea what this all means to you. And Amy, you made an automatic assumption that this change means that he doesn't love you, and you believe you're being betrayed."

Amy nodded slowly in agreement. Casey just sat there.

Men's sexual requests can tap into some pretty strong reactions from women. We don't always understand where they're coming from. We are sensitive about being "used" or objectified. That's a nightmare scenario for women like Amy, and even myself, who grew up in love with love and see romance and adoration as a confirmation of our own specialness. It's a highly personalized interaction, a form of reverse objectification that's not primarily sexual. The man becomes a "love object."

Amy limited sex to an idea she had about "making love" and what she imagined that looked and felt like. Any other sexual expression was threatening to her and meant that she wasn't being loved. I couldn't blame her, given the history of how sex has been used to harm women, steal their power, humiliate, punish, degrade, etc. Sexual acts have been wielded as a power tool against women in so many ways across history and cultures, and much has been written to inform on this history, so I won't elaborate in this book.

Yet I mention this to make a point: There's good reason that some men's sexual requests bring up deep fears for women. I think women have been robbed of their own freedom to enjoy these very acts. Staying in the "making love" zone is a nice, safe, protected place. But it doesn't breathe, it doesn't grow, the life of it stagnates. Both sides end up feeling constrained. This really smacks of fearful control not love. For Amy and Casey, the dance of sex was not fluid, there was no exchange of creativity, no freedom to share spontaneous desires.

Truth be told, I don't think men and women necessarily have such different drives. I think both want love, and both want to fuck. Quite frankly, I think separating lovemaking from fucking is a false dichotomy. It's matter of perception. We have to look at the meanings we attach to various sexual acts.

Let me take a brief aside to illustrate just how a sex act can take on various meanings. Once in a while, I will transcribe a particularly riveting session in my notebook. Hank was one of those cases, and the moment he left my office, I had started writing.

Hank was on an intense, edge-of-the-seat, manic, anger-filled rant about his wife not giving him blow jobs. He wanted me to know, with every bit of his entitled rage, that he felt he deserved them. I let him go on and on without trying to stop and structure the conversation. I simply listened intently, silently made notes about his concerns, and occasionally gave him some validation as feedback. This diatribe provided some seriously rich material about his psychological landscape.

Hank: "Have you seen the Don Juan movie? That's me. I am a trained seducer. Does she know who I am? The women I can get? I had so many women and I fell in love with her, made the choice for monogamy, and now I'm like a stallion trapped in a barn!"

Me: "You're saying she doesn't appreciate what a great lover you are?"

Hank: "That's right. She doesn't recognize who I am. My skills are wasted on her. I should find somebody else who will appreciate me. [pauses] You know what? I want to be seduced. My wife is so passive, she just expects me to do all of the initiating. I give her oral all the time and she never gives it back! I have to ask her to give me a blow job, and let me tell you, it's a big chore for her. Like she's doing me a favor. She doesn't get it. It's like I'm dealing with an inexperienced teenager. This is so boring. I want the dance. Instead, she acts like she's tired or busy. So . . . what? Am I a burden to her? She makes time for everything else; am I not important enough? I am fed up with being ignored. I told her that she needs to start giving me blow jobs or we are getting a divorce."

Me: "You feel rejected by her."

Hank: "She betrayed my love. I gave up everything for her."

Me: "All the other women?"

Hank: "Absolutely. I treat her like she's a precious diamond. I adore her and give and give. I get nothing back."

Me: "So, what the blow job means to you is that she wants to value you. To adore you. To give to you."

Hank: "Yes. Right."

Me: "Sounds like you're giving what you want. Do you think she knows that a blow job represents all of this to you?"

Look at the meaning of the blow job for Hank. He equates his wife giving him a blow job with her valuing and loving him. He attaches love to sex, neurotically. And he thinks a blow job is his primary need, but in fact, his primary need is love.

Blow jobs *are* especially laden with meaning. They are often associated with subjugation and sometimes humiliation, or as a tool to get something—generally by the man—but the power can go both ways. But how about a blow job as a loving act? A giving act?

Anytime a patient is fervent about any sex act, I have learned he often has an issue with trust. He doesn't actually believe someone will consistently meet his needs.

When an emotional need is unconsciously conflated with a physical one, it becomes a massive rejection when that individual is told no. It feels so personal.

Hank had set up some unrealistic sexual expectations for his wife: If you give me blow jobs then you love me, and if you don't then you don't love me. But Hank just didn't see the distortion. Many men do this: They only see the sexual need and then blame monogamy when they are disappointed.

Another patient, soon to marry, reinforced this when he told me, "If I have to go from sleeping around with many different women, or at least believing that I have the option to do so, to getting married and only having sex with one person for the rest of my life, then the sex better be good."

Talk about putting pressure on a lady! However, in seriousness, men can become internally conflicted with these two competing desires: the many versus monogamy. But it's not like a battle where one side wins and the other is defeated, the "many" slain forever and monogamy the glorious victor. It's more like a perpetual race where one desire ekes out a slight lead while the other breathes ferociously down its back. Although the desire for love and companionship may win the competition, there is still that sense of entitlement that because *he chose her* to be his one and only, a magnanimous choice in his eyes, the life with her had better be good and worth it.

This thought process is a total mistake for men. When they deal with the intrinsic sexual dichotomy of one versus many by operating in fear, they set themselves up for failure. The quixotic guy quoted above was earnestly in love with his fiancée and said he was *happy* to make the choice to have sex only with her. But his pressure-filled expectation that he was giving up something, so the sex with his fiancée *better* be good, would only set him up for disappointment, because the expectation was demanding and irrational.

No sexual relationship is good all the time. And if anybody wants to tell himself the story that the single life is more glamorous, and that being married will lead to boredom, then that is exactly what he will find. Guys who put this pressure on their lovers are often the least skilled in the seduction department.

Guys with sexual egos based on the number of women they've slept with tend to have the hardest time with monogamy, not to mention the grandest sense of entitlement and the most false ideas about their own sexual prowess. One patient told me that one night when he was in the mood and his wife was not, he felt so frustrated and angry that he said, "Do you know how many women want me?"

The actual answer to that was "none."

Many men are afraid that a relationship means leaving the realm of boundless opportunity, only to get lost in the dreaded matrimonial apocalypse: the sexless marriage. They picture the "end times," only with no rapture, no savior, no heaven. They have been left behind. Meanwhile, everyone else, all the single guys, are out there getting it on.

That fear makes sense. This is about men losing their vigor, their life force. As one of my friends told me, "Sex is life."

That's right, I thought, and in a very fundamental way. But also it's an existential matter. Sex drive is about expressing that one is alive, vital, and creative. The concern men have about being trapped in a sexless marriage is not because they are simply biologically oversexed creatures. The death of sex in marriage is not, as some in my profession posit, simply a fear of death. Rather, the death of sex in marriage is a *real* death, a death of spirit, a death of hope.

It would probably surprise Amy to learn a truth I discovered from many of my male patients—and it surprised me as well: The topic they're most frequently interested in during sex therapy . . . *is love.*

However, it can be hard to see that because their feelings of love are often mixed with other seemingly contrary impulses that arise during sex—like aggression and fear—these impulses confuse and often frighten these men. They worry: Will I lose my power, my control? Their thoughts veer: I hate this overwhelming need for approval. I feel dependent, and I hate it. I hate her power over me. Am I good enough for her? Forget it, she's trash. Or on the masochistic side: I want to be dominated and taken over. It will make me feel safe.

It seems to me that a counterintuitive approach would be more productive. Abandon the idea that men and women have completely different sexual natures. If men and women could recognize the "other" in themselves, they could begin to make it okay for them explore sexuality as a couple.

I half-expected a call from Amy soon after our difficult joint session, and that instinct was right. She wanted to see me alone. She felt depressed about herself and couldn't shake it. "I thought I was the perfect girlfriend," she said. "Now I'm not so sure."

Amy settled into the couch and led off with a surprise. She had used Casey's computer to find the porn sites he visited, hoping to discover what had so enchanted him and why she "wasn't enough" for Casey. What she discovered was beyond what she'd imagined. "My first impulse was to compare myself to the women and pick them apart: their faces, their bodies, their clothes—what little they wore. But the more I looked, the more absurd it seemed. I actually started laughing. And then, well . . . I got aroused—and mortified—by sex scenes I'd have refused to do if Casey had asked. And then I masturbated."

Amy had experienced Casey's world, and it confused her. "Porn repulsed me *and* turned me on," she said, pinning me with a look of intense uncertainty. "I want to know what that means. I have to know."

I'm not entirely surprised that Amy was aroused by watching porn even though mentally she wasn't interested in what she saw on the screen. The body and the mind can be discordant for women.

This reminds me of a fascinating study in which sexologists showed footage of a variety of sexual acts to groups of men and groups of women hooked up to a plethysmograph, a device that measures blood flow—a sign of physical arousal—to the genitals. Both groups saw images of heterosexual sex, male and female homosexual encounters, a man masturbating, a woman masturbating, a handsome man walking on the beach, a woman doing calisthenics in the nude, and bonobos—a species of ape—mating. Everyone was asked if the footage turned them on—and the answers were then compared with the plethysmograph readings.

What men said turned them on was congruent with how their bodies responded. Straight men experienced increased blood flow when watching any images of women or heterosexual sex; their bodies did not respond to observing other males. Gay men responded to male homosexual images.

However, the women's results were entirely different. Their bodies responded to everything, even the footage they stated did not turn them on at all. They responded to straight sex, male homosexual sex, the woman doing exercises, even the bonobos!

This study certainly seems to indicate that female sexuality is much more expansive or, as the Chinese say, inexhaustible. The famous sex researchers of our time, Masters and Johnson, said that a "woman's capacity for pleasure would put any man to shame."

I knew what had turned Amy on, so I asked what had repulsed her.

"The pictures were offensive. Animals, underage girls, grandmas, women being treated like dirt. Seriously, what the hell is wrong with people? I can't imagine doing what I saw on there."

"What would that mean to you?"

"I don't want to put myself in some degrading position for his pleasure," she said with a disdainful emphasis on the word "his."

"I can see why that would hold you back from wanting to do anything erotic," I said.

"Erotic? The fact that he gets turned on by this filth makes me incredibly mad."

The idea of herself as an object to be desecrated upset Amy. I could understand that. She wanted a man to see her body as sacred and her sharing it with him as a gift. I felt the same and worried sometimes that the soul of sex had been lost. Amy and I were both daughters of socially conservative parents who didn't talk freely about sex, who preferred relationships locked into what we were led to believe would be a never-ending euphoric stage—despite what we sometimes saw with our own eyes.

Amy hadn't moved on. Instead, she often found herself going along with sex play Casey initiated in order to work on the relationship. And now Casey opening up about his desires had played right into Amy's fears of being only for "his pleasure." There is often deeper meaning to the roles of giving or receiving pleasure. Amy had a choice here about how to perceive the role of giving him pleasure, but first I needed to understand what this meant to her now.

"What makes you mad about it?" I said, remaining exploratory and decidedly nonjudgmental.

"Like he wants to disrespect me," she said, her furrowing brow and intense eyes signaling that she was sinking deep into a contemptuous rage beneath her controlled surface.

"What's bad about that?" I said, trying to escalate her.

She gave me an angry look for asking this question, as if the answer should be obvious, but I was simply leading her to the core of her anger.

"I want him to love me," she said in a soft voice.

"So it's important to feel loved. And when sexual activity starts to pull away from what feels like a loving tone, that threatens you?"

"I like 'normal' sex. I like when he wants to make love."

"Of course. Yet some of the porn did turn you on . . ."

"Yes . . . and I don't understand why."

"It means that you have a preference for sex with a very romantic tone, but maybe there *is* room for you to expand your experience."

"I am not doing anything degrading," she insisted.

"Amy, you're still reacting to what you saw on the Internet," I said. "I don't blame you. But are you willing to consider that the Internet isn't the *only* resource for eroticism?" Perhaps Amy would respond to the same suggestion I'd made to Casey.

"I don't know."

"Let's try the most important resource: your own mind. Maybe there's a way for you to have an erotic experience without feeling degraded."

"How is that possible? What do you mean?"

"You get to be erotic, yet you stay connected to your love. A lot of what you saw online is designed to be salacious and outrageous in order to get attention. Most of it follows very basic male sexual scripts. How about developing *your own* sexual script, one that puts you in a position where you get to feel good about being erotic."

Amy asked what she had to do. "Some reprogramming," I said, gently. "But first, all this aside, do you believe that Casey loves you?"

"Yes. I guess. I mean, if it wasn't for the . . ."

I cut her off. "So, yes."

"Yes."

"Then first you have to move beyond using sex to validate that you're loved. You can assume it because you already know that you are."

"I guess. Yes."

Amy still looked confused. "What I mean is forget what men want. You will be more of a turn-on to Casey if you know what turns you on. I know, 'making love' turns you on. But you thought it was the only thing that turned you on. Now you know better. So what fantasy do you have, would you indulge, *in addition* to making love, especially because you know that no matter what Casey wants, he's not simply using you; he loves and respects you."

Amy asked to start seeing me individually, and, after consulting with Casey, I agreed.

I learned more about Amy as the weeks went by. She was thirty-eight years old and had lived in a rent-controlled apartment on the Upper East Side for fifteen years. She'd earned a business degree in Dallas, Texas, but suddenly decided to move to Manhattan—few of my patients were actually *from* New York—to pursue a career in fashion. Her parents didn't approve, but it was nonetheless a turning point for her. Amy started a semi-successful career working as a freelance stylist for various catalogs. Contrary to my first impression, she was a happy, chatty girl's girl, always experimenting with her clothes and a range of avant-garde ensembles and accessories. Whenever she came in, I had to take a moment to absorb the visual feast or else I would be too distracted by her bold, mismatched fabrics or her large, anachronistic earrings—and we'd waste precious session time with mutual flattery about the cuteness of each other's outfit. She could have easily been one of my girlfriends, and I had to remind myself that she was a patient.

Amy was psychologically savvy and revealed that she was obsessed with self-help books. Casey, however, liked to joke that although she had a library full of advice, she never put it into action.

Although Amy was a woman who clearly cared for her physical appearance, it wasn't for sexual purposes; she was more an animated piece of art that enjoyed being viewed and didn't want to be vulgarized by the "cheapness" inherent in sexuality. Amy was really a bit asexual. My challenge was to teach her to become a sexual being who could transcend the limitations she'd placed on herself and, by default, Casey. Freud talks a lot about how we constantly suppress our sexual instincts. Well, I thought, if we're capable of suppressing them, then we're capable of increasing them. If it's a matter of perception, then it's a choice. One can learn to sexualize anything or anyone.

This may have been a lofty idea for Amy, but I decided to start in a very basic way: cultivating her sexual energy. We all possess it, even if only a dim flicker obscured by the frenetic pace of our bodies. The energy of sex is all around us, like a great current that runs through everything. Sometimes relaxing is all we need to do to feel it, but often we need to see it as well, to perceive it. There is the obvious: sultry music, a soft fabric, the glow of a candle, poetry. Beyond that, there is the skill of attuning to a life force greater than one's ego strivings; an ability to luxuriate in the senses and to develop a fine appreciation, that of a connoisseur or an artist, a cultivated eye that can see the beauty in anything, in this case the *sexuality* in anything. The rolling hills of a Moroccan sand dune had done it for me. As had a small motel room in the Southwest, intense conversation over wine in a French cafe, Cirque du Soleil in Montréal, a muddy riverbank, a seedy jazz bar, and a graveyard in New Orleans. The Gulf of Mexico at night in the heat of summer, when the water is about eighty degrees. A New York salsa club, being turned and dipped to the ground by anonymous Latino men, so fast that you don't know what's happened until the song is over, and the guy moves on, and you stumble away dazed, smiling, with your hair all tousled.

We use our bodies throughout the day for so many utilitarian functions that it's easy to lose touch with our physical self as sensual. I tried to explain to Amy how to connect, but it's not cerebral or abstract, it's visceral. So I took half a bar of dark artisanal chocolate—flavored with hints of cinnamon and chili pepper—from my desk drawer.

"Take this." I said, handing Amy a square, for a very basic exercise. "Now close your eyes. Breathe deep and take a bite of the chocolate. Don't chew. Just hold it in your mouth. Savor the texture and press it up with your tongue on the roof of your mouth. Can you taste the spicy pepper? Now swallow the chocolate and stay with the aftertaste. Notice how the cinnamon flavor emerges. Breathe in the cinnamon smell and shift your focus to your ability to make each part of your body come alive and experience pleasure."

Amy did as I asked. "Now, stay with me. Inhale and then softly exhale, imagining your exhale going through your vagina.

Gently squeeze your vaginal muscles and imagine your genitals coming alive. Again. Notice the sensation and relax into it. Again. Now, I want you to say to yourself, just in your head: 'I have the right to feel pleasure. I have the right to feel pleasure.'

"Notice what, if any, images come up for you. Allow your mind to drift to any scenario of you experiencing pleasure."

Amy's breath quickened slightly.

"Now repeat this to yourself: 'I am a sexual being.' Imagine yourself embracing and enjoying your sexuality, your right to feel pleasure. Notice what that looks and feels like. Okay, open your eyes."

Amy's eyes were wet.

"How was that?" I asked, mustering an encouraging smile.

"I forgot how angry I was at Casey. And I can't believe that I've never stopped to think about what I want," she said.

"Good. I want this to be about you feeling empowered instead of threatened."

In order to reduce her resentment toward Casey for his entitlement to pleasure, I wanted her to build her own sense of entitlement, and the first step was to give herself permission. If she succeeded in getting comfortable in receiving, then giving to him would feel less like a power giveaway.

"How often do you think about sex during the day?" I asked Amy one afternoon.

"Ha. Never." Interesting, I thought. How could sex get so shut out of her daily life?

"Would you consider an experiment?"

"Let me hear it first." Amy was still cautious about sex.

"To intentionally think about sex for at least three minutes, three times a day. You can do it anywhere—on the subway, walking down the street. I want you to notice the sexual energy all around you."

"In the grocery store? Produce can be very erotic," she said jokingly.

"Yes. Anything can be sexy. So allow sexual scenarios to enter your mind. Don't judge them, just start to notice what comes up for you. This is designed to get you in touch with your own sexual imagination."

"Okay, I can try it."

Casey continued to come in separately as well. Although his episode in Washington Square Park had helped him get in touch with his right to his desire, Casey still had work to do. He was still unable to share all of his erotic thoughts with Amy, because he was afraid she wouldn't approve.

I asked him to think about why Amy's approval was so much more important than his needs. A relationship isn't about making sure you have your partner's approval all the time. Sometimes you disagree or don't approve, but you still love each other.

Sex is a vulnerable place. We're sensitive to somebody saying, "Eww," or "That's weird and disgusting." But we have to be willing to tolerate that judgment, because the act of sharing is more important to our own integrity.

Not only do I constantly ask patients, "What do *you* want?" but I tell them to be who they are. I believe we have to honor ourselves first and be completely authentic even in the face of disapproval. Otherwise you're selling fool's gold, and the lie is eventually uncovered.

Casey and Amy had started out at opposite poles, with Amy focused on expressions of love and Casey looking at pornography. Those look very different from the objective outside, but what they had in common was that they had both been hijacked by social constraints. I had been trying to guide each of them through a morass of social messaging, personal symbolism, and emotional meanings to get into the clearing. I had needed to see Amy alone so she would be less reactive about Casey's proclivities than if he had been sitting there, too. I could keep her focused on herself instead of on him, and I was careful to frame my interventions as self-growth. But my goal was to guide them both back toward each other as they each took a personal journey through almost a year's worth of sessions.

"Did you come up with a sexual scenario?" I asked Amy the next time I saw her.

"Yes. At first it felt like a chore, an assignment to think about something, but it ended up being fun. I did it for longer than three minutes, three times a day. I felt like I'd discovered a whole world around me. I ogled guys at the gym, imagining them with their shirts off. I signed up for a judo class—all that wrestling around seems sexy. I went for an art gallery walk, and some of the paintings, with their fiery colors, seemed full of sexual tension. I even flirted with the checkout guy at Trader Joe's.

"And I initiated sex with Casey—which I never normally do. I used to wait until he wanted it."

"How did Casey respond?"

"He liked it, and I even noticed that over the past two weeks, he's more affectionate with me."

Casey had already told me how he had responded to Amy, and that her willingness to embrace her sexual side helped bring out his loving side. "You're doing great work, Amy. You seem very excited about your sexual development," I said.

"I am, too," Amy said.

The Amy that Casey had raved about in his first session had become more and more present. She was bright, enthusiastic, and engaged. I enjoyed her.

Amy's choice to put effort into her fantasies gave her a new sense of vitality. Casey's reaction to her was simply a pleasant side effect. As for Casey, he felt more warmth for her than ever. And increased lust.

Another notable side effect: He had much less interest in his nightly porn habit.

MARK

I was really beginning to enjoy practicing psychotherapy with men, except I noticed that after a few sessions, I kept having this sense that I was useless. If I could sum up the theme of the hour it would be the man saying, “It’s fine. I got it. I’ve got the problem all solved.” Yet his body would totally betray him. I’d notice a constricted jaw, a racing knee, or a furrowed brow. I could tell that the man on my couch was feeling *something*, yet holding back, his body literally fighting against a revelation. Sometimes, while they’re telling me how great and fine they are, they’ll literally pinch their face or neck as if they’re squeezing the opening of a balloon. And obviously if you pinch the opening of a balloon, the air stays trapped inside. When this happens, I cannot move forward with therapy until I ask them what it means to have feelings and even more important—ask them to show me.

The very nature of therapy collides with men’s common beliefs about masculinity. So I stop and ask an important question,

"What does it mean to be a man?" This can be an awkward moment because, obviously, I am not a man. And yet, as someone who regularly works with patients to redefine masculinity, I see myself as sort of a man anthropologist—a "manthropologist" if you will—observing, taking notes, categorizing unfamiliar behaviors and classifying subspecies.

When I inquire about their reticence to express emotions, I typically get some version of this answer: "Weakness." They all want to be the Marlboro Man, I think. One notable exception was a young, stone-faced Bear Stearns banker who walked into my office and said in an almost robotic tone, "I want to learn how to feel. Can you teach me? I want you to make me cry."

Mostly, they defend their stoicism. My client David once said, "What are you trying to do to me? Women don't want a nice guy." Paul said, "I don't want to appear too soft. One shouldn't let a woman know how much she is loved."

When I suggest that the strong position is actually to allow and express the feeling, some of these guys look at me like I'm crazier than a nine-eyed billy goat (as my brother says), asking them to be unmanly. One patient shouted at me, "You're trying to make me talk like a girl," to which I replied, "What's the big deal about admitting to your feelings? It's natural. It's part of the human experience. It carries information about you." I know some men are tempted to discount this point of view because of course a *woman* is going to extol the virtues of feeling—but they know somewhere deep down that I'm speaking the truth. That said, I get that sharing feelings isn't functional in many of the competitive environments that men operate in—e.g., sports, business, the stock exchange floor. I get that a soldier isn't going to say "Hey, Sergeant, what you said really hurt my feelings," but when it comes to psychotherapy and, importantly, in their personal relationships, men can probably take the bulletproof vest off.

This weakness idea does not just apply to men crying or becoming sad. It often extends to other feelings, like insecurity, fear, and even love. Some men will inhibit their expression of love for fear they will appear soft and wimpy. The consequence of avoiding conversations about feelings can result in sex becoming a repository for a man's unexpressed emotions and unrequited needs. As a result, these men are searching for their masculinity through sex rather than bringing masculinity *to* sex.

To be fair, men fear the demonstration of emotions in part because this has real-world consequences. They believe they'll lose a woman's respect or, worse: the entire relationship. And there is some truth to that possibility, particularly sexually. I recently had a conversation with some of my friends about which male archetypes we fetishize, and everyone gave answers like police, firefighters, soldiers, even mafia types. Nobody wanted to sleep with Eckhart Tolle. One girlfriend told me, in the most aggressive tone I have ever heard come out of her otherwise sweet, feminine mouth: "Sometimes I just want to be manhandled. I want to be ravaged." These ladies wanted villains, vampires, and Christian Grey.

I think women are hungry to enjoy a man's masculinity. They want to feel his strength, both his biceps and his internal muscularity. When a man is super-focused on pleasing and gets anxious because he's so intent on his performance, he often appears obsequious—you know, "Is this okay?" or "What do you want me to do?" or "Did I hurt you?"

This doesn't sound like a guy who knows what he's doing. He's giving the woman control in that moment when she doesn't want control.

Turned off by a lack of confidence, a lot of women go looking for the alpha male and end up getting a jerk, a guy who takes and gives nothing back, who exploits and maybe harms them. That's not the kind of masculinity a woman wants either.

A man I know once told me that there are two types of men: the Gladiator and the Gardener. He said you get either the physically strong, macho, aggressive type who is great in bed but doesn't make much of a companion outside the bedroom. Or you get the Gardener, the sensitive, poetic type. He'll brush your hair and bring you ice cream when you have PMS, yet may not be so great in the bedroom. He'll make love to you, but not with the force and strength that demonstrates his masculinity.

Personally, I've never wanted either type. The pure Gladiator is powerful, but destructive. A pure Gardener becomes inert and impotent. But when the best aspects of both mix, then you have a man who can in his own way combine strength and tenderness. I think generally speaking (though these attributes aren't technically so gender specific), women are turned on by men who possess the ability to be decisive, to take charge, to know what to do; who embody that natural, testosterone-fueled sexual energy and express that in their desire for a woman. Finally, women love a man who exudes passion, which requires, of course, *emotion*.

So, typically, once we work through this "what it means to be a man conversation," giving my patients a safe place to share their feelings eventually opens the floodgates. Even though some of them give me a hard time, in the end they seem to really want it. They just needed permission. Nothing makes me more proud than some tough-as-nails guy from Queens telling me that he's "feeling more connected" to himself or that he's experienced a little sadness today. I say, "That's wonderful. Congratulations. You're a human being. You're able to feel, to love—and to say so. No freak-out necessary."

One of my more unforgettable patients was Mark. An affable transplant from Portland, Oregon, with an earnest good-natured charm, he was immediately likeable. Maybe it was his implacably pleasant and agreeable nature, or that easy smile that spread the smattering of freckles across his nose and cheeks, that gave him a boyish appearance despite his being in his mid-thirties. He was a single guy who worked as a staff writer at a magazine. When Mark arrived for our first session, he began with some awkward superficial small talk about the vagaries of New York and the latest pop-fiction novel that he had in his hand. I noted that he seemed to be derailing the start of therapy with his nervous chatter.

When I finally started to ask about the reason he'd come in—erectile dysfunction—Mark cut me off and blurted that there was something else.

"It's just that . . . that, I'm looking for a relationship, but if I tell a woman what I'm *really* like, I won't stand a chance." I waited, unwilling to interrupt. Mark seemed to desperately want to spill the truth; he also seemed horribly afraid. I couldn't imagine what he might be hiding.

"It's okay," I said. "This is a safe place."

Mark let go all at once. "I'm a sadist. I need to hit a woman to get aroused."

The incongruity of his sexuality and his acquiescent presentation made his words initially difficult to process. I sat there scanning this sort of Peter Pan–esque man sitting in front of me nervously fiddling with his book bag. He was wearing a graphic T-shirt and Converse sneakers, the kind of outfit that says, "I'm not corporate, I don't have to go to an office, therefore I don't have to look grown up." Not exactly the kind of guy who exudes the authority needed to pull off sadistic fantasies.

"I'm part of the city's underground S&M community," he explained. He said he had an elaborate collection of paddles and flogs and he patronized a midtown members-only sex dungeon just a few blocks from the tourist attractions in Times Square. "That's where I meet the women. We never engage on a personal level. I don't know where they live or what they do for a living. Usually I don't even know their real names. The only information I get is their sexual boundaries and preferences, and the 'safe word' to let me know if they want me to stop.

"But outside of that place I'm shy and I can't approach women," he said, looking humiliated.

I just want to pause for a moment to impart my general thoughts on the S&M community. They are adults in control of their sexual behavior, who define their boundaries, have a good time playing with surrender and the opiates that pain releases. This is much different from the men mentioned in previous chapters who want to dominate a woman they consider inferior, who want the woman to have no control or choice. That said, I always approach a client's sexual preferences with an attitude of curiosity rather than unquestioning acceptance, which I think closes the door on exploration and growth.

I was intrigued by this dichotomous creature who could easily have been the guy next door, an inconspicuous coworker or that guy you passed up for a second date because he was too nice. To really understand what was driving this man, I needed to understand exactly what turned him on. His sexual fantasies would give me clues to his psychological needs and unresolved emotional conflicts. I could see that he was uncomfortable and tentative with me, so I was decidedly nonjudgmental yet direct.

I asked him to be specific about what went on at the club, and whether he felt anxious there. "No, actually. Just the opposite," he said. "These are structured scenarios. I can hide and lose myself in the role-playing. I can be someone else."

"What kind of role-play do you like?"

"I like having the woman sitting up on her knees, hog-tied. Then I slowly circle around her, surveying her body. I strike arbitrarily with a flog somewhere across her back, buttocks, or breasts. I like to look at the redness on her flesh, the chill bumps across her skin, and her eyes beginning to water."

Mark's posture straightened perceptibly. "I like the look of fear in her face as she pleads with me not to hit her again. She makes promises that she will please me if I just let her go. She says she will do anything I want. I ignore her and create a delay between each strike so she builds fear in anticipation of the next. I really like when she begs for me to stop. But of course, it's all just a game and she really does want it."

"You like eliciting fear."

"Yes."

"And she's the one who's afraid, instead of you."

"Yes."

"What do you like about seeing her in pain?"

"It forces her into compliance."

"How do you feel about that?"

"Confident, in charge, in control, powerful."

A very interesting reversal, I hypothesized. I wondered if he was projecting his fear onto them, then his psyche was somehow attempting to overcome that fear by dominating it.

"And then you have sex?"

"Rarely," Mark mumbled. "I know, I know. It's strange. But even though I get hard during the foreplay, I always lose my erection."

The fact that he was losing his erection was an interesting piece, but I chose to hold off on exploring it for now. "Okay, so it seems we're getting some information about what you would like to feel around women. See if you can connect this to any of your relationships. . . ."

"Outside of the club I think of myself as sensitive and even romantic, and I guess I find women intimidating," he said, a bit embarrassed.

"In what way?"

"They're hard to please. My last girlfriend, Kathy, was very domineering. I did so much for her and she was really unappreciative, and the more I did for her, the more demanding she became."

"What did you do for her?"

He rolled his eyes as if to say, "What didn't I do?" "Here is an example," he said. "She had a dog, a devilish little Chihuahua named Rudy. He was so nervous he would pee anywhere, all the time. Kathy put one of her super maxi pads on him, tied on with a pink headband. One time Rudy got out like that and she made me chase it down Houston Street."

I stifled a laugh.

"Look, I know I am a pleaser," Mark said, making the observation first as if to fend off an imagined critique. "I do it at work, too. My boss is a ball-buster, and I am constantly working extra hours and taking extra assignments from her. I never complain. I'm just like the horse in *Animal Farm*, a worker eager to please the boss."

I now had a loose idea of at least two sides of Mark's life—and there might be more. But how did they mix? "What was sex like with Kathy?" I said. "Did she know about . . ."

Mark cut me off. "She had no idea I was into the S&M scene. I could tell that she wouldn't be into it, so I never suggested it. So we mostly did what *she* wanted. *We made love.*"

Another familiar refrain, typically brimming with resentment at what my patients believed were narrowly defined female parameters for "good" or acceptable sex.

"How did that work for you?"

"Actually, it was pretty good," Mark said, grudgingly, "but lots of times I lost my erection right before sex."

Hence the stated reason for his visit—which didn't sound "pretty good" to me. With this opening, I could have jumped into an exploration of Mark's ED, but I wanted to delve into his bifurcated and compartmentalized life. "So, you kept a significant part of yourself hidden?"

"I guess." He paused, recalling something. "But we did have a houseboy scenario that we both liked. I would walk around Kathy's apartment in my underwear and she would command me to wash the dishes or sweep the floor. She talked like a drill sergeant, and as I followed her orders, she would distract me during my task by gently stroking me and saying 'good boy,' in a soft tone."

Whether at the S&M club or in the world outside, Mark's sex life was themed with obedience. With anonymous women he was in charge. With Kathy, she'd been in charge. Although Mark felt powerless outside of the club confines, he had eroticized his powerlessness. But something didn't make sense.

"If Kathy liked the houseboy scenario, what stopped you from telling her about your other fantasies?"

"She was always so judgmental. I didn't want to upset her."

"What was it like for you when Kathy was upset?"

"She got angry and insulting, then she refused to talk to me," he said, wanting to move along. "So I'd avoid upsetting her." I noticed that Mark was clenching his jaw.

"I am sensing some resentment."

"Oh no. No, no. Not at all."

Mark had just given me my chance to reflect his answer back at him. "Oh, so you *enjoy* self-sacrificing?"

Suddenly Mark had no answer. "It sounds like Kathy ran the show in your relationship," I said, pushing harder.

"Well, I'm not selfish," he said, defensively. "I take pride in working hard and being a giving person. I have always believed that these are important principles. I have a very developed sense of justice . . ."

Mark went on, pontificating about the virtues of service to others. I had tapped into some rigid barricade that made him feel superior. Although I didn't yet know what it was, his justifications were a clue that he was protecting himself from *feeling* something. Perhaps it was the anger I could sense leaking out from behind the smiles, contagiously irritating me. I imagined that under his consummately polite and self-righteous façade, Mark just really wanted to rip someone's face off.

After we said good-bye, I realized that despite my irritation at the end, I had—curiously—enjoyed my session with Mark. Mark interested me. He had an earnest, good-natured charm, peppered with wit, and generally seemed like the quintessential nice guy. Ironically, that was possibly also part of his problem, and why he couldn't keep an erection, I thought. Penetrating a woman requires aggression. Perhaps Mark had an unconscious conflict with aggression that in real life trapped him in a passive role.

Zeroing in on Mark's passivity reminded me of what a girlfriend had told me one morning as we walked in Central Park. She'd just started dating a new guy. She was very excited, all in bloom. He seemed like one of those perfect-on-paper guys: good-looking, successful, super-smart, interesting, polite . . . check, check, check. But his flaw was that he couldn't make a decision on his own. She explained that simply trying to set up a date could be an exhausting process.

"He wants to know what kind of food I like, what restaurants interest me, what side of town is best. Then he'll call to make sure a reservation time is convenient—even though I've already told him I have the whole night open for him.

"Why doesn't he just say, 'I made the reservation at this restaurant and I will pick you up at eight'?" she complained. "Just take charge!"

"What's he like in bed?" I asked jokingly. The look on her face said she hadn't gotten that far—and had now begun to wonder as well.

"What should I do? When I tell him I'm happy to let him decide, he gets kind of annoyed."

Rami was also that way sometimes. "Once, Rami and I were walking on the Lower East Side looking for a restaurant," I told her, "and he kept saying 'Whatever you want.' I thought, if I hear that one more time I am going to scream. I said, 'Rami, just tell me what *you* want!' and he said, 'I don't care, whatever *you* want.'"

"What did you do?"

"I did the first thing that popped into my head: I yelled, 'Make a decision right now or I'm going to leave you in the street!' and I started walking away."

"Did he?"

"He grabbed my elbow and pulled me into some random Mexican restaurant two doors down. I hated the food, but I was happy."

That weekend, in the taxi on the way to the airport to visit Rami, I scooted forward in the backseat and looked through the sliding Plexiglas window at the driver's taxi license.

"Hey, Mohammed, are you married?"

"Yes."

"So, who has more control in your relationship? You or your wife?"

He laughed. "My wife controls everything. *Um krone.*"

"*Um krone*? What does that mean?"

"A woman with a horn. This is the word we use for a woman who has her foot on the head of a man."

"Is that a good word or a bad word?"

"Oh, that's bad, a very bad word."

"Figures! Come on. What's so bad about letting the woman have the control?" I said, taunting him.

"It is wrong for anybody to have all of the control," he said. "There is an old Arabic proverb that goes like this: Call someone your master and he'll sell you on the slave market."

It didn't sound so bad to me to be a woman with a horn. But I also wanted my man to have a horn—pun intended. The energy shifting back and forth, both partners able to hold on to their own strong sense of personal power; the battle itself creates just the right tension for sexual passion.

Mark arrived for his next session and made the usual aimless small talk as he settled into the corner of the couch and pulled a pillow protectively onto his lap. He glanced at me expectantly. I gave him a little smile but didn't say anything. Neither did he. I noticed that Mark's passivity elicited the controlling side of me, and there was a pattern developing; the more he yielded, the more I took over with my agenda. I was sure that he was drawing this response out of other people as well. I decided that we needed to address this dynamic, so I intentionally took the passive role. I could sense his unease with the silence, but I kept my mouth shut as we both looked away and then back at each other.

"Did you know that there is a hole in the wall right by your desk?" he said.

"Um, hmmm," I said, not bothering to turn to look at the hole.

"You're quiet today, Doc."

"I'm just waiting for you to begin," I said.

"Isn't that *your* job?"

"You want *me* to decide what we should talk about?"

"Isn't that what I'm paying you for?" he said, with a tense smile.

"You're paying to have someone tell you what to do?"

"I don't know what to talk about today."

"Okay. I'll wait," I said. I laid one hand in my lap and carelessly twirled a strand of hair with the other, but never took my eyes off of Mark.

"I don't think I'm getting anything out of this," Mark finally said. He angrily reached for his shoulder bag, an implied threat that he was ready to walk out.

"You seem upset with me," I said, purposely stating the obvious.

"Just sitting here staring at each other isn't going to help me," he grumbled.

"Well, you're paying a lot of money to work on *yourself*," I said. "I'd think you'd be more proactive about it."

"I feel stuck," he said.

"I understand," I told Mark. "You're used to being told what to do by the women in your life. I thought that you didn't like that."

"You're right."

"Then why are you asking me to tell you what to do? Do you see that you're getting angry at me for not directing you? On some level, you *want* someone else to be the leader. If I do it for you, then what will you learn from me?"

This was an uncomfortable maneuver on my part, as well,

because I hate the silence and inactivity. They bring up my own fears of being incompetent, my need to say or do something. Of course, I also didn't like my patients to get mad at me, but this technique usually worked.

I let Mark think about that. Meanwhile, I wondered if his desire to have someone else take responsibility stemmed from a significant childhood incident. I asked, and given some direction at last, he explained that his father had died suddenly of a heart attack when he was twelve years old. His mother's grief had unraveled her. She'd become severely depressed and was barely able to make it to work, let alone raise her two boys.

Mark was the oldest and painfully aware of how badly his mother felt. He didn't want to do anything to upset her further. "I just wanted to make her happy," he said. To that end he helped around the house and stayed out of trouble. He also cared for his little brother and made sure he didn't upset their mother either. When his brother did, Mark meted out the discipline. "But I never got angry."

"So, you took on the good boy role?" I said strategically choosing my words.

"Yes."

"Did you get a chance to go through a rebellious stage?"

"No, I couldn't, I was focused on keeping Mom happy. I couldn't disagree with her or disobey her."

"What would've happened?"

"She was so fragile and anxious. I couldn't stand to see that. I would've felt so guilty so I stayed in the good boy role and tried to be proud of it. My brother was the one who got to rebel, and I hated him for it."

"Sounds like you're still in that role with women now."

"Yes, with my ex-girlfriend and at work."

"What's the cost to you?"

"What do you mean?"

"What are you like because of this role? What's happened to you?"

"I don't speak up for myself?" he said. "I . . . I let women walk all over me?"

Mark had nailed it. "You aren't willing to be disobedient, to get angry, to just go out in the world and get crazy."

Ironically, Mark's problem couldn't be solved with traditional sex therapy techniques because the genesis wasn't sexual. Mark's childhood situation had caused a rupture in his personality. His desire to be responsible was overdeveloped, while his desire to be independent lurked in the shadows and came out only when he used his sexuality as a prop. His fantasy world compensated for what was missing day to day, but it also got in the way of what he really wanted in a relationship.

My goal was to help him integrate his worlds, so I needed to focus not on his sexual behavior, but on him accessing the anger toward his mother. Maybe then he could find a more consistent sense of personal strength instead of the role-played pretend strength that he enacted in the dungeon.

Mark was comfortable asking for what he wanted if the woman wasn't important to him. And yet, in a relationship, he was obsessed with keeping his girlfriend happy at the expense of what he wanted. As soon as a woman became important, he regressed to an old dynamic between himself and his mother. I thought he might be unwittingly projecting that anger.

"So, when you don't get what you want, let alone ask for it, you blame it on the woman and get angry at her."

"Most of the time, I don't even know that I'm angry. I just get irritable and depressed. And I never let her see it until, like I did with Kathy, I decide I want to break up. That was two years ago, and I still feel guilty. She looked so hurt. She was still in love with me." Mark paused. "Why did I do that?"

"You needed space because you aren't able to be yourself. Suppressing anger and other spontaneous self-expression leads easily to irritability and depression."

"Maybe that's why I felt so free after I left her. I wasn't even heartbroken. But the guilt hasn't gone away."

"Now we see why it's so hard for you to get angry. Guilt is the emotion that blocks you. You're still protecting your fragile mother."

A memory flashed across Mark's face, and he told me a story. "She would sit at the kitchen table, not saying anything, just staring at a pile of bills. One time, my brother fell off his bike and had a big gash across his cheek. My mother saw it and started to cry, then she got angry. She grabbed him. She had that look in her eyes of being out of control, unraveling. I panicked and stepped in. But I've never forgotten that image."

Feeling so responsible for his mom's stability had been a heavy burden for Mark to carry.

"Who was your rock?" I asked.

Mark shrugged. "I didn't have one. So I found what grace I could by keeping her happy. Keeping the house clean. Keeping my little brother in line. When she stopped crying, she would smile, and then everything was okay and I could be at peace."

"Your whole sense of stability was wrapped around keeping her happy. Did that mean that you didn't always get to express yourself?"

I felt certain that the anger underlying Mark's passivity would be the golden key, that moment in therapy that unlocked the door and allowed him a personal paradigm shift and access to his strength. People often think anger is a negative emotion, one to avoid for obvious reasons, but anger is one of my favorite emotions because when you tap into it productively, it indicates a sense of self. It signifies that rights and boundaries have been trespassed on, and that they deserve respect. Mark was blocked, and I needed to enable him to hold on to his love for his mother and, at the same time, access his sense of self.

Using the famous "empty chair" technique from Gestalt therapy, we pretended that his mother was sitting in my office. I asked him to face her in that chair and tell her everything that he really felt as a teenager. I backed just out of his view, interjecting occasionally to gently reflect back what he felt. As usual, I tried to intensify his emotions. "Tell her all the reasons you're mad," I instructed. Mark struggled for a moment to say anything, and his first few words fell flat. "Come on. Tell her what *you* needed," I urged.

Suddenly, Mark let go. "I needed you to stop fucking crying and be a parent," he spat. At that he recoiled slightly, perhaps attempting to contain a wave of emotion ready to burst. But it was too late.

"Tell her what else you needed," I said, softly.

"I needed you to see me, but you were too consumed with your own grief. Why couldn't you get yourself together?" he shouted.

"You were so angry at her," I prompted.

"I felt like I didn't even exist. You forgot about us. You weren't there." Red-faced and shaking, he leaned toward the vision of his mother. "I had to do *everything*. I had to be the father." Mark clenched his fists. "I was trapped. Fucking trapped."

I say that I like anger, yet when I actually sit in the room with a man's raw, unbridled rage, quite frankly, it scares me. The more upset Mark became, the more I hoped he didn't lose it completely. On the other hand, he *needed* that anger, and the worst thing I could do was short-circuit it as he himself had for years. Even more, he needed *a woman*—me—to be strong enough to sit with these feelings.

Mark's chest heaved. "Dad died . . . and you abandoned me, too."

Mark's grief had finally risen past the anger, to the surface. He covered his face with his hands and turned away from me. All I could see were his shoulders convulsing and the sobs of unrestrained tears. After a time, I handed Mark a pillow and told him to hold on tight. To watch someone grieving was incredibly moving. I didn't want to cry along with Mark, but there was no way to remain detached. I choked up.

Now that Mark had finally begun to liberate his anger and grief, the question was what he would do with this powerful experience. Would he overcome his guilt and use his anger and grief constructively, or would he close up again and revert to familiar patterns? Would he be able to claim his own voice? Could he seize the opportunity to finish becoming a man?

I had one more appointment that afternoon, then I went for a walk in Bryant Park. I hoped to find a chess game. I was contemplating terminating my relationship with Rami—again—but this time it would be for real, the final breakup, the Big One. I had begun mental preparations, creating a safety plan and gathering provisions.

I was replaying in my mind an evening just a few months earlier, following one of our many mini breakups, when Rami flew to New York unannounced and called me from a small Spanish restaurant in the East Village. He had that "I'm just in the neighborhood having a drink" attitude and asked if I'd join him. My heart raced, both excited and anxious, but I knew him well enough to tell that behind his casual tone, he actually wanted to see me. And that meant he didn't want to let go.

Even so, I arrived at the restaurant determined not to agree to get back together, only talk, share some dinner, some wine. Well, half a bottle of wine and we were drawn together again through our mutual reverie about the life we had wanted to share. He took my hands in his and said, "*Habibi*, you don't have to work. You don't need to worry about anything. I will take care of your student loans, everything. We will travel at will, you can write or do whatever makes you happy."

What a proposition! I felt that familiar warm euphoria. We held hands. I never thought I would be free from working, or my student loans. I came from a middle-class background and had always expected to work hard. In truth, I had never completely believed that Rami's lifestyle could be real for me, yet his promises appealed to my deepest wishes to be saved, rescued, taken care of by this handsome, older, benevolent father figure. And together we would live in carefree joy.

"I also want you to work on your Arabic in case we want to stay in the Al-Bireh house for a while," he said.

Now I was manic with ideas, practically panting at the ornament of my dream life dangled before me. I had visions of hookahs and Arabian jasmine and all the places I wanted to go. I wanted to explore the entire Middle East—Tunisia, Lebanon, Jordan. Yes, I would be a modern day Freya Stark, famed travel writer and early female explorer of the Middle East. To travel anywhere, anytime, to pursue any creative endeavor? Who wouldn't take a chance on this opportunity? I thought. I saw nonprofit work, a book, a documentary. I wanted to go to Brazil and Tanzania and Greece. And at the time, I was particularly obsessed with a small town in central Mexico, called Guanajuato, a former colonial silver trading outpost famed for its beauty and celebration of romance.

I wanted the exotic, extraordinary life. Maybe we could make this relationship work. Somehow.

"Our home base will be in Florida," Rami said.

My stomach muscles knotted. This again. A loaded declaration. Rami recognized the look on my face.

"Rami," I said. "You *know* I don't want to live in Florida!"

Rami laughed. "Don't worry. You'll never be home."

Leave New York? No way! It was quite possible that I was more in love with New York than with Rami. I didn't want to go home to Florida. I didn't want to leave my friends, my career. I was happy, satisfied. I recognized there was a great cost to this offer: everything I currently had. If I accepted, would I be gaining everything or losing everything?

Now, as I sat in the park, I thought about the dinner we'd had the night before. Rami sitting across the table, quiet, his eyes staring at some point over my shoulder. He showed almost no interest in what I had to say about travel, politics, my work, his life. It was like talking to a carrot. I wondered if I just bored him. Did he know my stories so well by now that he couldn't even fake interest? I felt like a favorite old dress that I'd had for so long that I could no longer see its beauty despite its timeless quality.

All of the tumult seemed to have taken its toll and my worst fear was coming true. Our passion was waning. Further, Rami was stressed and preoccupied. The economy was crashing and he was losing a lot of money in his businesses. It would have been easier if he had just told me, but that wasn't his style. Rami withdrew into that clandestine closet deep in a man's psyche, that little "situation room," where men go to solve all the world's problems, alone. And in true macho fashion, he didn't want me to see that he was bordering on despair. However, his eyes were wandering again, and I had never felt so invisible. With each breakup, we would come back together, largely connected by fantasies of the future. There would be a brief period of euphoria, drunk on a cocktail of our own imaginations, only to wake up a few months later, hungover and staring flatly at each other over pasta.

I knew that I had to let go of Rami. That night, alone in my apartment, I began to realize that the loss of the dreams seemed more daunting than the loss of the man.

All I had to do was figure out if I could create my dream life on my own.

One day Mark came in thoroughly depressed. This was actually a welcome change from his consistently pleasant façade. When I asked how that felt, he said, "Hard. But it feels good to just be real. I've also been speaking up at work and it is so liberating."

"That's a big step!" I was proud of him. Mark *had* been slowly asserting himself in all areas of his life over the past few months. I wanted to support this new authenticity and told him so. "It's easier to feel connected to you. Closer. This will help you in relationships."

"Well, while we're on the subject, there's something I have to tell you," he said, suddenly energized. "I have a crush on you."

"You do?" I said. That was all I managed to come up with. I was flushed and a bit stupefied, but I wasn't completely surprised. I had sensed something in the air, and to be completely honest, I had a slight crush on him as well. We'd been working together for many months, and I looked forward to our sessions. Once, I caught myself checking my makeup before he arrived.

Did I cause this? I thought. God, I hope I didn't do anything to encourage a crush. Was I subtly flirtatious? I rifled through my memory searching for moments that I might have been mildly flirtatious. I did feel more connected to him than most of my other patients; the conversation was more natural at times than therapeutic. I decided to keep it focused on him, not me.

"Tell me more about these feelings."

"I feel like you get me."

My stomach fluttered involuntarily. "That sounds like a new experience for you. What is it like for you to have someone really try to understand you?" I asked.

"I have never felt so seen or cared for. I've never had a relationship with a woman like this. Not even my mother."

I had been a strong female figure for Mark, able to draw out his anger with a calm, guiding hand—something his mother couldn't do because of her own grief. I had heeded the words of a former mentor: "Always provide the patient a sense of your internal muscularity; your strength itself is the intervention. People instinctively respond to that. It makes them feel safe." I had created a protected place for Mark to let go of his role as the dutiful son and unfold as a human being.

"Yes, this is a powerful relationship," I explained. "You like that someone can see you, the real you. And I accept you unconditionally. This is what you are looking for in your life."

I hoped that Mark would understand that his crush actually stemmed from the basic nature of the successful therapeutic relationship: that I actually knew and accepted his innermost being. I'd always been struck by how hungry people are to be heard in this way. That was my job, but this wasn't something special about *me* specifically. Mark had no idea who I was outside of the office, or about my own romantic travails.

"I feel like a fool for telling you this," he said, averting his eyes. I hated to see him embarrassed.

"Your honesty took courage," I said. "I respect that."

"I wish that I could do this with the other women I meet," Mark continued. "I went out with a group of friends from work this weekend and I ended up talking to this girl. I actually initiated the conversation, which is new for me. She was really smart and interesting; we talked all night and left the bar together. We walked back to her apartment and we kissed in front of her door. Then—and this surprised me—she started fondling my crotch and asked me to come upstairs. But I said no. I could tell that I wouldn't be able to keep my erection."

My first reaction was a flash of jealousy. Then relief that he had changed the subject to another woman. This was exactly what he needed, to start meeting women in regular social settings. I had to stay clinical, almost mechanized, to fend off this unfamiliar personal reaction I was having. "The great thing here is that you connected with somebody and you initiated. When it became sexual, that's where your anxiety kicked in, so let's take a look at that."

"I liked that she was aggressive. I liked that about her personality right away."

"Why?"

"It takes pressure off of me."

I told Mark that I thought he needed to face that pressure instead of avoiding it.

"Okay. Well, then, I've been having a sexual fantasy about you," Mark said, abruptly.

Oh no, back to me. Was he thinking of spanking me? Now, uncomfortable or not, I had to hear the content of his fantasy and use it therapeutically.

"All right. Tell me about it."

"I don't know . . ."

"You obviously want me to know something," I said, a little thrown off, even made nervous by this new assertiveness with me. "You don't have to give me the details. Was there a theme?"

"Warmth, soft touches, hard kisses. I imagined you in my apartment, lying in my bed, our bodies locked together."

"How did you feel in the fantasy?"

"Turned on by my own tenderness for you."

"I want you to think about what that desire says about what you need in your life right now." To my delight, Mark made the leap.

"That I'm capable of loving feelings and getting turned on at the same time?"

This was real improvement. Love had taken up residence in

Mark's fantasy world and he had become more assertive in everyday life. Along with his newfound confidence, he seemed less angry. The air in the room was lighter. His smiles weren't a lid for a cauldron of rage. Mark was a legitimately happier guy.

When Mark stood to go, he walked toward the door more slowly than usual and paused by me, contemplating something. I smiled and said nothing. But my cheeks pinked and I fantasized about him pinning me against my door, kissing me. I moved behind my chair, unconsciously protecting myself from my own fantasy—and, God forbid, transparency. This was so unusual. I had never thought of any patient this way, and believe me, many attractive and interesting men had sat on my couch, some of them insatiable flirts. And yet I'd never been attracted to any of them.

Mark walked past me with a lingering glance and left me alone, to stumble around my office, feeling disheveled and undone—and guilty—as if I had actually done something very wrong.

As I reflected on that session, I recognized that I had just witnessed something beyond the simple crush that can occur in any therapeutic relationship. I realized that a major shift in Mark's personality was being acted out in his relationship with me. He was transforming from this sort of divided passive-aggressive man into one who was assertive, bold, and courageous. He wasn't a Gladiator, or a Gardener, he was becoming an integrated man.

Mark took a risk to share with me how he felt, and I was inspired by his revelation. Courage, I thought, is necessary to sustain a relationship. Mark was exhibiting a quality that I myself couldn't quite conjure in my own life. I loved to breakup with Rami or at least fantasize about breaking up, instead of facing down our issues directly. I couldn't, however, walk away from my patients. I had to stay with them and provide them with a sense of unconditional acceptance, and it was this very process that drew out of me a new strength that I hadn't ever known with a man. I'm not talking about a stand-by-your-man, codependent type of philosophy; rather, it's about having the courage to take bold action instead of seeking the cowardly self-gratification that makes one feel safe. It's easy to decide that you want a relationship because you enjoy companionship or being loved, but the act of giving love requires risk and a tolerance of uncertainty.

Intimacy requires bravery. Mark allowed me to see his desires, probably knowing that he would be rebuffed, and I wished I could give him some kind of medal of valor for that. So many of my clients can't follow through with real change in their sexuality because they have difficulty exposing their erotic desires. Why? It brings up self-doubt, fear of rejection, and fear of being different or weird. This is why the work of sex therapy often becomes about overall self-confidence, because this is what's needed in order to handle intimacy. Mark's disclosure to me was a step toward self-acceptance and ultimately toward a relationship for him.

When I think about the ideals for masculinity, they are in essence the same ideals for any relationship to be successful. Talking with men about what kind of man they *wanted* to be in a relationship helped me to identify the important questions women should ask themselves when looking for a man. How does he deal with emotion? Can he manage anger and sadness, or will he blow up or stuff it down? Will he act out and attack, or withdraw? How does he deal with stress, because life is full of that, and women should know that the man with whom they share their lives can make it through with them. Can he be comfortable with love, with giving *and* receiving? Can there be mutual support, each being the other's rock and safe place? Can he maintain his love when she frustrates him and things are difficult between them? Can their love not be the place where they lose themselves and their individual voices, but the place where they find them?

I remember expressing concern to a friend of mine that at the outset of my private practice I really wanted to help women, but primarily I was working with men and wondered if I had lost my original vision. "You are helping women" she replied, "more than you realize." I thought carefully about my role in helping to shape the way my patients related to women. I frequently encountered variations of the Gladiator-esque cultural conditioning of masculinity, even in the seemingly mildest mannered of men, and I saw it as a real obstacle to their personal growth. I was determined to play a role in redefining what it means to be a man. I wanted to help men access their own natural softness as well as their internal muscularity. I wanted to help them redefine what it meant for each of them uniquely to be a man. I thought about what an ideal man is to me. He remains steady in the face of love's uncertainties; he remains steadfast in the face of a woman kicking and screaming, threatening to leave. He handles his needs for power in an honorable way; he uses his power to build and create. He doesn't become powerful by taking from others (particularly not from women), but through sharing and giving. He finds it through being a helpful force in the world. He works to facilitate the greatness in others, including his woman. He has the utmost respect for himself and the person he loves. He does not see the successes of others as a threat because he is firm in his own value. He does not need to exploit others' weaknesses in order to build his own strength.

Getting these guys, and me, to put these ideals into action wasn't easy. When I was frustrated about my patients, I would call my mom and tell her I wanted to give up. "Why am I helping this person?" I would ask in moments of contempt. She once told me to look up Corinthians, chapter 13, in the Bible. "Read the first line." I did. It was "Love is patient." Boring, I thought. Next.

Wait, that is my problem. I was actually struggling with my ability to love. Love wasn't easy at all, not like romance. It wasn't just a warm feeling; love required a certain toughness, an internal fortitude. I'd come to understand that men are frustrating and imperfect. They don't live their lives to be exactly what we want—and if they did we would probably hate them for it. The truth is, no man is my savior, my Jesus, my Buddha, or my mama. He is just a man.

When it comes to tolerating intimacy, we all have our own thresholds for how much we can actually withstand in a relationship. Rami and I were all over the place. I would move close, he would pull away. I would pull away, he would move close. Nobody liked to be the closer. We both wanted to be pursued. He would open toward me, then start a fight. I would feel vulnerable, then start a fight. This was all born out of insecurity, not passion. Nobody was being brave or bold.

I wrote a lot in my journal during my affair with Rami, mostly confused lists and endless pages about my search for clarity. At the core of my ruminations seemed to be the question "Does he really love me?"

But the real question was "Am I capable of love?"

Just like David had asked me about himself.

Patience, courage, tolerance. These are the qualities that determine the answer. Because I'd asked this very question of my clients and helped them answer it for themselves, I began to really learn the lessons of what the skill of loving actually is. They were the much overlooked, less glamorous parts of love.

Mark reported that he'd lately made fewer visits to the S&M club and spent more time with female friends. Reducing his use of the "dungeon" was never a goal of therapy because I am not in the business of trying to reform someone's sexual routine unless it's causing a problem. But therapy had helped Mark become more assertive beyond its confines, and that obviously had rebalanced his needs. The more powerful he felt, the less he seemed interested in flogging women—though he admitted that this would always be a part of his repertoire of sexual turn-ons. But now he just wanted to find a loving relationship.

Our next few sessions were unproductive, and filled with idle chatter but no emotional depth. Neither of us spoke about what had happened between us. I could have invited him to discuss the impasse directly; I knew what to do when I sensed resistance. But I chose not to. I wanted to avoid the conversation because in the back of my mind I knew it would also be the last time I would see him. Mark broke the silence.

"I have real feelings for you," he said, confidently. "This is not just me projecting some fantasy onto you. Believe me. So I have a question I want you to answer without psychological interpretation. Stop being my therapist and just be you."

"What's the question?"

"Do you feel it, too?"

I wanted to say no. I wanted to lie, but I didn't want to steal the truth from him. Authenticity was what I promoted, and the truth was that I did feel something, and I didn't want him to question his intuition.

"Yes, but . . ." I stammered. "This is a one-sided relationship, Mark. Do you think you *really* know me? I don't think that's possible."

"That's bullshit. I *do* know you, Brandy. I may not know where you live or where you came from. You don't share anything about yourself, but I know the look in your eyes, and the way you smile, and your warmth, your intelligence. I know it well. I've known you for a year. You can't hide yourself."

I was totally thrown off guard. He was right. I felt something. What was it? I wasn't sure. Maybe I was flattered. Possibly, he was tapping into my own deep hunger to be seen. My patients rarely tried to know me, typically only asking about me to ensure my qualifications to help them. Most of what they knew of me was based on their own projections. I felt as if I—the real me, the woman behind the psychotherapist—was becoming invisible. While I encouraged their authenticity, I was busy burying my own, laboriously concealing my moods, my true thoughts moment by moment. I may have been bored, tired, worried, or full of exuberant joy, forcing the smile from my face in favor of the implacable serious attention needed to create a safe container for them to unfurl their tears, their fears, their despair. I carefully tracked every subtle flicker of emotion expressed in their bodies, attentively extrapolating the nuances of their verbiage—their tone, their choice of words—microscopically searching for their core and mirroring back that which even they could not see in themselves, while my own radiance was eclipsed in their formidable dark shadows, there in my small dark room.

I longed to walk in the sun, share my stories, reveal little bits of myself. Sometimes I'd tell a story about that morning's subway ride, the play I saw the night before, or a book I'd read. But when I did, I was often met with a hurried placation, a message that psychologists are not to use up customers' paid time to chat about themselves.

Therapy is largely a parasitic relationship. Some days I felt used, resentful. Mark wanted to know *me*; he had chiseled away at my façade, and his attention sent a new energy coursing through my veins, reanimating my limp spirit like water for a withering plant, bringing me back to life. I had never experienced this before. I wanted to reveal myself to him, and it made me feel guilty.

I couldn't interpret this away like I did with the other patients who came on to me or to other women they encountered, like David. With them, I used a rehearsed strategy of reflecting back the way that they related to all women. This was all new for Mark. He was taking a real risk and he was earnest. I wanted to be super-careful with his feelings.

"Yes, Mark," I finally said. "I do have some romantic feelings for you as well, but it's not appropriate for me to act on those feelings in any way."

"I think that's ridiculous," he said. "People meet in all kinds of places; therapy happens to be the context where we met. Are you saying that if I met you somewhere else this would all have been different?"

"Sometimes we find connection with someone we can't have."

"I checked out the psychology regulations," Mark countered. "After two years, we could be together."

"Mark, I would never consider a romantic relationship with you. Working with you has been very meaningful to me, as you know, but my role in your life has been to help you grow. This is only a temporary role."

That was my final session with Mark. We both agreed that it wouldn't be helpful to work together anymore. I said that I would have to refer him to someone new. I recommended a male therapist on the Lower East Side. I knew this was the ethically appropriate protocol; I'd just never imagined I would ever be in that position.

Truth is, Mark's pursuit of me was in some ways a success for him. His ability to speak his truth was admirable; there was a bravery in his vulnerability, a resolve in the face of my rejection. It was all downright sexy. The look in his eyes was resolute. I was looking at a new man. He seemed strong, powerful. I had rehabilitated him into the kind of man I admired, the kind of man I really wanted.

I thought carefully about my reaction to Mark. After the initial, difficult stage, our conversations were often effortless. I felt a sense of twinship, the ease of a familiar soul. I was looser and lighter in his presence, as if even though I had to conduct sessions and always remember my job, I *was* somehow myself with him.

Mark was not exotic. He was a salt-of-the-earth, middle-class, middle-America guy, of average appearance, average wealth, and average intelligence. There was no room for projection, no sparkling fantasy to color around him, no promise of far-flung adventures. The interaction felt clean, wholesome, pure in its affinity. I saw him as a real person and I felt pure enjoyment in his presence. Mark taught me something important about what I was missing: a connection based on the real man, not based only on what I needed from him, not based on what I wanted him to be or thought I could change him into. This interaction was simply two real people enjoying each other for who they really were.

And yet, even as I was drawn to Mark, I was disturbed by how much he was like me. Just as I held up mirrors to my patients, Mark had been inadvertently—but tellingly—my mirror. I saw myself in him, a disavowed part of myself, the simple girl from a small town in Florida, and what I imagined to be the mediocre, vapid, dead life that I had wanted to escape. However, in Mark, I saw a beauty that helped me to lift that faulty perception and embrace reality.

A couple of weeks later, Rami called. "I booked us a flight to Mexico," he said. "That place you've been talking about, Guanajuato. . . ."

BILL

Patients are often circumspect when meeting a therapist for the first time, and I was used to being tested during the initial sessions. I think of the exchange as similar to what happens when going on a date: Sitting across from each other at a romantic restaurant, the potential couple are both asking themselves, "Can we connect? Are we a match? Will we have a good relationship?"

Bill, however, didn't want to wait. "Before we start, I need to know what you're gonna be like," he said, leaning back, arms folded across his chest. Court was in session and he was ready to judge.

"You're wondering if I'll be able to help you?" I said, raising my brow and smiling.

"That's right."

Many questions are aimed at figuring out if I'm truly going to be helpful or not. I've heard questions about my work history, what school I went to, or if I've had any personal experience with a patient's problem. The answer may not be what he wants to hear, so I've learned to be agile. "I'm a single woman, but I've successfully treated married couples. I don't have children, but I've treated mothers. I treat men with erectile dysfunction, but I don't have a penis. I may not be able to identify personally with your life circumstance, but you're paying me for a specialized set of skills, not similarities."

On rare occasions, I've been judged even before speaking. Once, an elderly woman walked into my waiting room, and when I opened the door to greet her, she took one look at me and said, "Oh, no," and immediately walked out. I followed her into the hallway and asked if she'd come inside and tell me what was going on. She agreed, and said that she didn't believe someone so young-looking could help her. Fortunately, she let me explore that further with her, and it turned out that she felt ashamed of asking for help from someone younger than herself. She ended up working with me, and once she got over her initial resistance, it went well.

But with this guy, Bill, his incredulity with me was far greater than the average; it was as if he started with the assumption that I would not be helpful or available to him. He seemed like a needy guy who expected no one to meet his needs. I was in a position of defending myself before we even began.

"Tell me what you need from a therapist," I asked.

"I don't want someone who's just going to sit there and nod her head for an hour," Bill said.

"So you just want some direct guidance?"

"Yes, but I'm still not sure about you." Bill looked me over, appreciatively, then said, "Maybe I should have gone with a male therapist. You may be too distracting for me."

"In that case, I may be *exactly* what you need." I told him that if I'm eliciting a reaction, then who better to address that reaction?

"Yeah, maybe," Bill conceded, with a chuckle. "You're not my type anyway. Okay. I need a lot of help. Maybe I should come in every day."

Another test: this of my availability.

"You're pretty urgent about getting the help you need," I observed.

"Well, I'm a sex addict. Do you really know what sex addiction is like?"

His challenges were beginning to irritate me, but I reminded myself to be patient. "Why don't you tell me what it's like for you," I said.

Bill gathered himself and explained. "Here's what it's like for me . . . I love tucking my kids into bed. Love watching them drift off peacefully while I read to them. And yet that deep love is mixed with anticipation about what I'm going to do after they're sound asleep. You would think I should feel guilty for what I'm about to do, but I don't. That doesn't come until afterward. All I can think about in that moment is what I want."

"And that is?"

"The rush of meeting someone new for the first time. I love the feeling of driving out of my neighborhood, past all of the quiet suburban homes, and heading to the Bronx. It feels dangerous and adventurous."

"You're looking for a rush."

"I never know what's gonna happen. I feel like I did when I was a teenager and cruised around the city with my friends on a Friday night, looking for a thrill of any kind. Maybe we would pick up girls or get in a fight or find our way into some exclusive nightclub. Yes, I like the high. The anticipation. But sometimes the ritual of getting it all set up is more exciting than the real thing."

"How does that make you feel?"

"Disappointed. It's anticlimactic. So, I look for more until I get what I want."

"More what?" I asked.

"More women. I can go through four or five a night. The most was ten in one night."

"That's hard to believe."

"Are you judging me?"

"No, just surprised. The number sounded impractical. So that's possible?" I smiled. I was also a bit surprised that I felt no contempt, no disgust or desire to poke at his fragile defenses. I was calm, but not numb. I realized that I could tolerate what Bill had said and remain focused and engaged and connected to my empathy, without drifting into my own reverie. I was right there with Bill, and I felt this mix of kindness and my own internal strength. This was a state I had always understood I was supposed to embody, but right now I actually felt it.

"Yeah. But I'm not necessarily having sex with them," Bill explained. "And if one pleases me, I'll stay with her. You have to understand that I'm very sensitive about what you think about this. Don't get me wrong: I have everything. I've been fortunate in business. I have a beautiful wife and I love my children more than anything. But I feel restless, antsy. Kind of like, Is this it? Shouldn't there be more?"

Bill was a semiretired real estate investor in his early fifties who'd cashed out at the height of the market. He lived in Connecticut and worked in Manhattan, at his leisure. For fun, he played golf and talked to prostitutes online. He always wore super-bright-colored Ralph Lauren sweaters of hot pink, red, or canary yellow. His whole demeanor was kind of lackluster, only his rainbow-colored sweaters suggesting some inner flicker of light. Bill knew pleasure, but not happiness. I think he was befuddled to discover that the lifestyle he was living and had long aspired to, the proverbial "good life," which involved the daily gratification of all of life's big and small pleasures, had failed to produce actual fulfillment. I had seen this before and thought, This is the dilemma of the man who doesn't need to work. There is no more challenge, nothing to conquer, nothing to create. Instead, his unstructured days gave him freedom and all of the existential crises that go along with it. Bill in retirement lacked dreams and aspirations. He didn't have much reason to get out of bed in the morning. Nothing really lit his fire; he had no passion, no drive, no purpose.

Then he hit an unexpected wall. Bill's accountant told him that he'd spent half his previous year's income on his extramarital adventures. Panicked, Bill sought advice and a friend recommended me.

"This money thing has really gotten out of control," Bill said. "I used to be able to keep it contained, but not anymore. How am I going to hide this from my wife?"

"How much did you spend?"

"Two hundred thousand."

I involuntarily winced.

A couple nights later, at dinner, I told some girlfriends that I had a new patient: a sex addict. Maybe it was the wine, but they convulsed with dubious laughter. "Come on," Margaret said. "Is this for real? Guys have been doing this since creation, and now, suddenly, it's a mental condition? Isn't this just pathologizing normal male behavior?"

"Yeah. It's just an excuse to justify doggery," said Jane. "This is the pop-psychology diagnosis du jour so these bastards can get off the hook. Now we're supposed to feel bad for them. Poor men; they just have this unfortunate disorder where they can't keep their penis in their pants!"

"I think I'm a sex addict," deduced one of my roommates. We all paused to look over at her.

"Yes, confirmed," we said, in jest and truth, remembering that the night before she had brought home yet another guy and failed to ask his name until they were in the cab.

"Do you seriously feel bad for them, Brandy?" Margaret asked. She'd recently been cheated on.

"Well, in this case I can find empathy for the guy," I said.

"Then maybe you should start a charity for these poor tramps," she said.

"I'm not suggesting that you pity men with sex addiction, or excuse their behavior. Or justify it. Or forgive them for the damage they've done, if it's not in your heart. I'm just saying that they are ill, fallible, and deserving of compassion—at least in my office."

I wasn't surprised by these reactions. Sex addiction was still a developing field of study. That diagnosis—not formally listed in the DSM, psychology's diagnostic manual—was still being hotly debated.

However, the behavior is clearly real, and there is a big difference between sex addicts and womanizers. Sex addicts are usually ashamed of their behavior and feel out of control. They're often depressed. Womanizers feel fantastic, and in control. I noticed that womanizers seek out ego gratification, while sex addicts seem to be searching for something else.

Sex addicts lose all sense of proportion and control, engaging in compulsive sexual activity with life-destroying consequences, such as draining a bank account to pay for sex services, masturbating so often that they bleed, or losing a job for obsessive porn-surfing on the company's dime. They suffer the repercussions—and they still can't stop. Over time this behavior can develop into a physiological condition exhibiting the same neurological changes that occur in the brain of a substance abuser. As with any addict, the brain's ability to sense pleasure becomes stymied. This is also known as "pleasure deafness." The pleasure threshold changes, becoming so high that the addict needs more and more sexual encounters to experience pleasure. So, if the emotional reasons behind this behavior aren't convincing enough for the doubters, the addiction becomes further entrenched by a physical need.

I try to guide these patients to be more aware of the actual nature of their desires. I want to make the unconscious motivations conscious. With men, in particular, a whole host of emotional yearnings appear to weave into what they want, even though they may not know it or admit it.

Bill confirmed to me that he needed more and more sexual encounters to get the same rush. The craving consumed his thoughts during the day, then distracted him from spending time with his wife and kids in the evenings. Sessions at his home computer turned quickly into reading emails from the women he met online. "I have to open them," he said, helplessly. "If I ignore them, I'll just obsess. So I end up chatting online, maybe masturbating. Then I arrange to meet someone at the end of the day—as long as I think she'll do what I want."

"And what is that?" I asked, following Bill's lead.

"I want her to be dominating, but warm and loving at the same time. That's a particular mix hard to find in a prostitute."

"I imagine so," I said. His dilemma sounded awfully familiar.

"I want her to take control and know what I want, to know how to place my head on her breasts, kiss my forehead while she strokes my cock. I want her to whisper to me in a nurturing tone, tell me to relax, that she will take care of me." Bill's voice quivered with embarrassment. "A lot of these women don't want to do this. They look at me like I'm a . . . creep."

Say what you will about Bill's condition, but I didn't think he was creepy for wanting to experience this aspect of femininity, even if it was mixed up with sex and prostitutes. His need was beautiful actually.

"Prostitutes are all about the transaction," Bill complained. "There's no real seduction. They don't get it. They want the money up front, no kissing and no affection. I have to weed those out. Sometimes I can find and pay for what I want. Yet it still feels mechanical. I can go through several tries a night."

"And this satisfies you? You feel fulfilled?"

"Not really. It ends when I get tired. Trying to get a prostitute to be loving is like trying to squeeze milk from a stone. I usually feel pissed off about how much money I spend. I feel like a sucker for all these fucking bitches!"

Bill's undertone of rage concerned me, but I set that aside because I didn't want to deflect what he was struggling to let out. Instead, I reflected back his frustration. "So, you're looking for a loving interaction from women who just won't give it to you."

"Yeah, I guess. I'm looking for some warmth . . . yeah, that's it exactly. I never put a label on it before, but that's it. I never knew what warmth felt like so I didn't even realize that's what I was looking for."

At that moment, this man twenty years my senior seemed like an unhappy infant whom I wanted to console. That surprised me more than anything, this desire to be nurturing after hearing a story about infidelity—a topic that used to evoke my barely contained disgust. I asked him to tell me more.

"You're disarming," he said, as if he had just realized something for the first time.

"Why do you say that?"

"I can't believe I am sharing all of this with you."

"I'm honored, Bill." And I meant it.

"I feel . . . exposed."

"You *are* exposed. What's that like for you?"

"Uncomfortable, but you put me at ease."

"I'm glad. And I'm glad you're allowing yourself to feel uncomfortable and still open yourself to me. *This* is courage, Bill."

My compassion for Bill lingered after he left. I had tears in my eyes thinking of how open he had been with me. I straightened the couch, cleaned my teacup, and locked the office door for the night. This must be what maturity feels like, I thought.

Something about Bill really roused some primitive feminine response in me, so I asked him to tell me about his mother in our next session. He described her as a self-absorbed alcoholic. "She had parties and boyfriends and always looked glamorous and happy and I felt like I was in the way. The next day she would always be hungover and would lay around the house in her nightgown and get angry if I disturbed her." When he felt really bad, he'd go to his mother's closet, take out a long satin nightgown, and use it to comfort himself.

Bill's mother took care of his daily needs but kept their interaction to a minimum. "No real affection, guidance, warmth, or . . ." Bill stopped abruptly, perhaps habitually, in the same way he had to in the past when his needs were unmet and he knew it was futile to try and get his mother to respond. Instead, he told me about how he'd recently gone to his childhood home and wandered around the empty house as all the old feelings came to the surface. The loneliness. The sense of being on the outside looking in.

"My wife isn't particularly warm either, but we have great chemistry and a good intellectual connection," he said. Bill deflated as he heard himself say the words. "She's Russian, though," he added, as if it explained away her temperament.

"How is sex with your wife?"

"Great, actually. I probably hound her for too much sex, but we do have sex at least four or five times per week. It's very physical, not very emotional. I used to complain and want more sex, but now I just leave her alone."

"Looks like a pattern here."

"Of finding women who are just as cold as my mother?"

"Of trying to make an emotionally unavailable woman show you some love."

"How am I trying to make them . . ."

"You pay prostitutes to give you something that most of them don't want to give you, and you're angry about it."

"Well, at least they get the domination part right."

"Actually you're dictating to them exactly how to dominate you, meaning that you're the one in control. What do you like most about being dominated?"

"I just want someone else to take lead and tell me what to do. But gently."

"Is that what you needed from your mother?"

"Yes."

"So, you have this frustrated need for a maternal love."

Bill's desire to be dominated was not masochistic; he wanted parenting. But his need wasn't so literal. He wanted the *essence* of a mother, those feminine qualities that both genders possess, but that we associate mostly with mothers: caring, nurturing, and assurance mixed with an internal fortitude. Although Bill made enough money to be virtually retired, in matters of relationships he was homeless, insolvent. I felt sad that he couldn't satisfy a need so basic to human existence. Without these feminine proffers, we are all without a home in the world.

"I need that love. It's intense. I can't get enough," said Bill. "Maybe that's why I push my wife for so much sex."

We'd finally arrived at the point where his messages had gotten mixed. Why would a man who wanted love seek it sexually? If you're thirsty, do you eat a sandwich? If you're tired, do you drink a glass of water? Here's yet another case of how men learn that it's *not* okay to be emotional, but it *is* okay to be sexual. Therefore, communication of needs, and their hope for satisfaction, happens sexually.

This really muddies the waters. Instead of sexuality being a free expression of love, life, and eroticism, it's weighted with other expectations. Bill's attachment of love to sex had become neurotic. This "high libido," "I just love sex" explanation many sex addicts give is really dependency masked as desire. What we have is emotional neediness, someone who wants to be reassured that he's loved. It's like saying "Do you love me? Do you love me? Are you sure? I don't believe you. Tell me again."

Sexual addiction is notoriously known as an intimacy disorder. I've read research reporting that 78 percent of sex addicts hail from families classified as "rigidly disengaged," which, translated from psychology-speak, means that there is profound disconnection and they feel chronically alienated. The afflicted are like buzzards, harpies, vultures, endlessly scavenging for scraps. They will eat anything. Women pick up on this neediness in men and are turned right off. Prostitutes and porn creators make serious profits from this. Unfortunately, in a marriage, this devouring insecurity is hardly erotic. Some women will go along with it in a man, however, and still have sex out of a sense of obligation because of their own co-dependency. Bill's wife was like that. She thought that if she complied with all of his sexual requests in the wake of his voracious need that he would never cheat on her. Little did she know that her strategy would not work with a sex addict.

I went on vacation. To Guanajuato. Yep. I went with Rami. Maybe it was because we were visiting the most romantic city in Mexico, a city so romance-obsessed that nightly ballad singers stroll for hours up winding, alley-like streets, singing love songs as people in the town follow, drinking wine and singing along. They end the walk at the alley of kisses, where people celebrate the act of kissing. This was my kind of town. If there could be a town soul mate, I finally met The One. I wanted to get married in the grand Spanish colonial church with the pink dome, in the center of town. I forgot, of course, about my big breakup plans, and we entered into the most calm and stable phase of our entire relationship.

Rami had even filed for divorce, of his own accord. I was astonished. I had come to accept that his and his wife's agreement to separate instead of divorce was solely financial. His decision to divorce meant that he was about to take a major financial loss, and I knew how much this had to mean to him, given how hard he had worked to build what he had. His story was one of those fabled tales of an immigrant realizing the American dream. He grew up in a refugee camp and came to the United States on a plane ticket that was given to him on a loan that took him a year to pay back. He arrived to New York with sixty-seven dollars in his wallet and moved into a two-bedroom apartment in Bay Ridge, Brooklyn, with eight other guys. He worked hard as an employee at a Manhattan deli and saved his money until he was able to buy his own deli with one of his coworkers. They bought a store, fixed it up, and made a profit that was more money than Rami had ever seen in his life. Years later, he owned many stores and properties. He no longer had to work, but he continued to carry the same wallet and always kept sixty-seven dollars in it, to remind him, he said, that at worst, he would break even—which was a good reminder, given that he might be even more impetuous than me. I understood the gravity of his decision and respected the sacrifice, the surrender, and the generosity in it. This was as a serious step for him toward trust in our relationship.

A few weeks later, Bill told me that his wife was suspicious that he might be cheating and had asked if she could attend one of our sessions. He also warned me that she thought psychotherapists were charlatans out to exploit people's sorrows for money. "I think she wants to make sure I'm really going to therapy," he said, "instead of seeing some other woman."

I encouraged my patients to include their spouses in the treatment process. I also wanted them to be honest, but Bill had fudged the truth already. He'd told Natasha that he was in therapy to treat a low-grade depression. It's tough enough to meet a wife, and more so when she doesn't know what's really going on. Some therapists won't even work with couples individually. There's no accountability when each patient gets to keep secrets from the other.

Natasha turned out to be a middle-aged woman whose dignified demeanor almost masked her nervousness. She wore a simple, starched, button-down preppy blouse and comfortable slacks. Her hair was a blond bob. I could tell she felt out of her element in the therapy office; she walked down the corridor of offices with a protective vigilance, as if she had entered a witch's coven.

Natasha forced a smile and offered a weak handshake as she carefully looked around my office and perched on the couch.

Although Bill's wife was dubious about the whole psychology enterprise, when she let her guard down, I sensed a basic warmth that didn't match Bill's chilly emotional assessment of her. Her rosy, fresh face seemed, in fact, kind.

Natasha didn't speak often during the first few minutes, but her eyes held an intense conversation with me. She'd scan me then avert her gaze toward Bill if I looked at her. Sometimes she'd look down her nose at both of us, then retreat, eyes vacant, lost in some thought. "Tell me what you talk about here," she asked Bill, softly.

"Depression"

"Is this helping?"

"Yes."

"You're so distant at home, if you are even there. You spend so much time away. Have you forgotten your children?" Natasha burst into spontaneous tears. I pushed the box of tissues toward her.

"I'm there every night to tuck them in," Bill said.

"Then you leave." She had placed her hand on top of his as if to hold his hand, but he wasn't holding her hand back. She was looking at him, with a look that said so much; it was the look of a woman who knows—and is begging to be told the truth; the look of desperate fear combined with a deliberate attempt to convey a kindness that would open him.

Bill looked quickly around the room. "I spend time with friends. I want to enjoy my retirement. I worked hard. Let me have this time."

"I don't have a good feeling about this," she said.

Then they sat silently, at an impasse. Bill offered no real answers and didn't respond to his wife's attempts to reach him. That moment was painful to witness. Intuition, this divine gift possessed by women, had now become a source of torment in the stolid face of Bill's lie, leaving Natasha confused by her own internal compass. She looked at me, with imploring eyes and a slight glance of contempt, as if she knew that I knew something and resented that he would he tell me, this stranger, this young woman, this therapist, everything that mattered most about the fate of her life. I couldn't stand it. I wanted to tell Natasha everything. But I couldn't. I was also angry at Bill for the collateral damage his selfishness had caused. I felt as if I was witnessing a woman's self-trust disintegrating, her perceptions stripped, the truth lost in hazy distortion.

Like some other clients who had been unfaithful, Bill did show guilt and remorse, and he had the insight and honesty to acknowledge that he was acting against his own value system. Yet that didn't stop his behavior.

I thought about how ordinary people get corrupted. It's a slow, insidious process that begins just outside of one's awareness, a soft voice that beckons for something is ignored while silently metastasizing until it becomes a powerful force, seemingly unbidden and intrusive, inhabiting one's bones and blood.

Swirling, the force occupies and moves the body into action against one's higher ideals, morals, and commitments, while loyalty to one's partner grows dim. The voice grows ever stronger, shouting, "I need" and "I want," as it becomes a blinding compulsion. Some are corrupted by greed, others by loneliness, envy, self-loathing, or jealousy.

Bill had been corrupted by his need for love.

I never knew what to expect from Bill when he came in, but I wasn't ready for the bombshell he dropped some weeks later.

"I think I may be falling in love," he said. "I answered a Craigslist ad and I showed up at this bar in the Bronx. In walks this gorgeous young Latino girl."

"Wow," I said.

"It gets better," Bill added.

One could only imagine. Had she been the gal to finally, willingly, dominate and nurture at the same time?

"I took her to this seedy motel in Yonkers," Bill continued. "When we got into the room, she told me she was a guy. Can you believe that?"

I was at a rare loss for words, so I just let Bill talk. We'd been at this long enough that he automatically answered all the "How did you feel about that?" questions I might have asked.

"I swear she was so beautiful, I couldn't tell. I would have been pissed off, but there was something charming about her. We kind of clicked. All we did was sit on the bed and talk for hours. She told me that she was only working as a prostitute until she had the money for a sex change operation. I encouraged her to go to school. I've been spending a lot of time with her: for sex, and sometimes just hanging out. I even give her a ride to her other johns so I can spend the time in the car with her."

Bill's face was incandescent. "What's different about this one?" I asked.

"Carla treats me as if she really cares about me. She listens, and she sees me in a way no other woman has, possibly ever. She told me yesterday that I seem lonely and lost. I didn't even realize it, but I believe she's right. There I am talking to this girl/guy, only twenty years old, sharing my angst about the emptiness of it all, and she gets it. I don't even care that she's a guy."

"She's really figured out your specific need," I said. What a brilliant maneuver. This prostitute gets that it's not sex Bill is looking for.

"I think she's really smart. I wonder, if she had been born in Connecticut instead of the Bronx, if she didn't have to worry about getting her ass kicked by the neighborhood kids for acting gay, I wonder what her life would have been if she had had the opportunity for better education or travel. You know, Carla doesn't know who Nietzsche, Steinbeck, or Proust is. She's never heard of President Roosevelt or even Trujillo, or the history of her parents' country, the Dominican Republic. She's never been out of New York, but I will tell you that she is so astute, so wise, I really value her opinion more than that of my own friends. If only her raw intelligence could have been cultivated in some way, how would her life have been different?"

Bill didn't know if he should refer to Carla as a man or a woman, if her behavior was real or an act. All he knew was that he had met someone he believed could *see* him, and it had brought him to life. There also seemed to be a theme in of all his Carla stories: He spent a lot of time trying to convince her to go to college. He couldn't believe that she had never considered the option of higher education. He started buying her books on history, literature, poetry. He'd buy her for the day and take her to cafes to read. It seemed that in Carla, Bill had found a purpose that drew him out of his existential doldrums. I had for months been trying to extricate him from a world where he felt lost and useless, bored and uninspired. Our abstract philosophical discussions had led nowhere. It took Carla to help him find some meaning in his life.

Bill planned to pay for Carla's sex change operation and provide her with a college fund. I wasn't sure how he'd accomplish that given his financial problems, not to mention Natasha and his children. Maybe the whole thing was just another manifestation of the addiction that had brought Bill to me originally, but I had a gut feeling that Bill's core motivations were shifting.

As Carla shared her experiences, she had pulled Bill out of the self-centered tar pit of his own yearnings and frustrations. Now he saw the world beyond Connecticut, golf, country clubs, and trips to Bermuda. The unfamiliarity woke him up to the bigger picture, and although Bill was dismayed to hear of Carla's struggles, he also had no impulse to turn his ear away from the grim truths she related. Instead he was reinvigorated, his mind suddenly fertile with solutions and ideas. He wanted to participate in life. Make an impact. Feel useful. Moreover, he was much less sexually preoccupied.

Now his mind was erect and potent.

Unfortunately, it wasn't long before Bill's excited frenzy to change Carla's life suddenly screeched to a halt. He arrived at my office in a panic.

"Natasha looked through my text messages and figured out that I haven't been exactly where I told her I went. Then she dug through my desk and found that I had secret cell phone and credit card accounts with charges for motel rooms, porn websites, and gifts. We got into a huge fight and she threatened to leave and take the kids."

I didn't want to be insensitive, but my first thought was, only threatened?

"Did you tell her what's been going on?"

"There's no way I can tell her the truth about everything," Bill stammered, undone. "I was so upset that I rushed out of the house and drove three hours to my mom's. I felt like I was having a nervous breakdown. But when I got there she wasn't home."

Bill clutched himself, devastated and once again feeling years of accumulated pain that his impulsive drive home had forced to the surface.

"I understand this, Bill. You finally reached out and once again couldn't find the mother that you need so desperately."

"Then I remembered the sexual abuse."

What? Why didn't he tell me about this before? I remained composed because I knew how Bill would react to any sign of judgment.

"I don't like to talk about it, but one of my mother's male friends molested me when I was twelve."

Bill seemed to collapse into himself, but I couldn't let him drift away. "What came up for you just now when you told me?"

"I wonder if I'm gay. I had sex one night with Carla, and now it's bringing all these memories back to the surface. When my mother's friend had sex with me, I think I might have liked it. I've been trying to figure this out for years."

"It must be overwhelming and confusing," I said. "Can you tell me what you liked about it?"

"The way he paid attention to me. He was very friendly, he took me baseball games. He was like the father I never had."

"That makes sense, Bill. You desperately needed a parental figure."

"I didn't really understand the sex part. I guess I knew it was wrong, but I was confused. He was friendly. He didn't seem like a bad guy." Bill pursed his lips. "Maybe I even kind of liked being touched by him. So, I don't know . . ."

"That isn't an uncommon response," I told Bill. "It doesn't mean you *wanted* the sexual relationship. Your mother's friend took advantage of your inability to fully understand. And even if you liked it, that doesn't mean anything about your sexual orientation."

Bill remained confused. "But I can't tell if I like sex with Carla because I'm gay or if I just enjoy being around her. I don't typically fantasize about men. I walk down the street and tend to only notice women."

Over time Bill determined that he had some bisexual tendencies that were partially caused by acting out this childhood trauma. And more than the sexual abuse itself, he was distressed that his mother hadn't protected him. In fact, she had allowed the abuser to babysit Bill and spend other time alone with him. Sometimes she would lock herself in her bedroom while straggling partygoers roamed the house, slept on the couches or the floor, and did drugs in front of Bill. This branded Bill's psyche in a powerful way. People often ask, "Why bring up the past in psychotherapy?" For Bill, it led to understanding the conclusions that he made about women in those formative moments. Bill's mother was inconsistent, so he learned to never fully rely on one woman. The whole idea petrified him to the point where he was unable to see that in reality his wife *was* very available, both emotionally and sexually. All Bill had to do was allow himself to receive what she had to offer.

Eventually I asked Bill what he really thought kept him from getting what he wanted—nurturing from Natasha. His answer sounded lame: "She's preoccupied with the kids."

"Sorry, but I don't buy that," I said. "She came to a session and tried to reach out to you. She is the closest thing to an *available* woman you've got. Come on. What's really blocking you from getting closer to her?"

"It's her," he insisted.

"Well, she's not here, so let's look at you. What do you imagine would happen if you were totally faithful to Natasha from now on?"

Bill confessed to a flash of panic and the fear that she wouldn't meet his needs.

"You mean you don't trust her?

"Well . . ."

"You didn't trust me either."

I believed that Bill's basic perceptions were twisted, as if he had looked into the fat/skinny fun-house mirror. "Your cravings for love are so big and distorted and the women are so skinny and withholding. This is where our work lies. These powerful fears and your desperate need for love. This is the legacy of the abuse."

Getting the insight can only take a patient so far. Once they learn to accept their relationship fears, the task becomes learning to deal with those fears. Only then can the transformation begin. It's a long process. For some, a life's journey. Recovery is about recognizing these fears when they surface, and practicing non-reactivity. It's a cognitive exercise. You talk yourself through it and breathe through the fear. Bill and I worked on this for months and practiced tolerating that unease as he took small steps toward reconnecting with Natasha.

As part of the process, he told Natasha everything, and the bold honesty—finally—allowed her to take steps forward as well. Bill also never spoke to Carla again, although he was grateful that their encounter had helped him to realize what was most important: that his life could take on a whole new purpose. Carla had inspired him to transform his existential emptiness into a passion for helping people. Bill decided to volunteer with an organization that helped inner city kids with preparation for college applications. And he did create a scholarship fund for Carla and a yearly fund in her honor.

In our final session, Bill had tears in his eyes.

"I want to thank you for how genuinely loving and compassionate you have been with me," he said. "No matter what I've told you, I felt accepted by you. You made me feel like a lovable human being. I want you to know that this alone is what has brought healing to me."

I wiped away my own tears and breathed deeply. I marveled at how of all the interventions I used, that the most effective strategy was simply to provide the patient with some genuine humanistic love. This was particularly pertinent for Bill because he had never been able to fully trust a woman. For me, I never had to go through the motions of empathy with Bill; my presence in the conversation was heartfelt and surely why the relationship had been healing. In psychotherapy this is called the "corrective emotional experience." In his or her relationship with the therapist the patient experiences new feelings that are so powerful that they break through the long-held assumptions, illusions, and conclusions about people and the world. But it's not change on a conceptual/intellectual level; rather, it's a change in the gut, a change born out of an experience.

The end result is hope.

THE EXIT SESSION

Reflecting on each of the cases written in this book, I realized that what was most enlightening for me about my first year of work with men was the dissolution of the myths that I heard women tell each other when trying to understand men. These fables reach such epic proportion that they seem true, even if somewhere deep down you know they are gross simplifications. First, there is the ubiquitous stereotype that men somehow separate sex from love. The cliché continues that all men want is sex, they want it all the time, and that the sex they want is solely genital-focused. Finally, there is the theory that all of this is caused by a biological drive in men to plant their sperm everywhere. Many of us simply accept that this is how men are. However, as I spoke with the men who were acting out these very myths, it only took a few sessions to reveal that men's sexual motivations actually aren't that different from women's.

It's not that easy for men to separate sex from love. I realized that love is such a central part of our humanity that we can't separate ourselves from the need to give and receive it. The need for love permeates everything we do, including sex. I noticed that the men who seek out disconnected experiences, anonymous partners, meaningless meetings in bars, sex workers, whatever, are still complaining that they want more passion, which differs from lust in its requirement of a present self. So this is where I'm getting it from, these ideas about improving intimacy; they are not my projections, they are straight from the dissatisfied mouths of men. They're asking for it. I think people want sex to matter, to be special.

I am not saying that sex should *always* be an expression of love, or that sex without love is bad or wrong. In fact, I just want to take a moment to say that I recognize that there are legitimate arguments to be made for the pleasures of disconnected sex.... There is an escape from identity and the ability to relish the purely carnal side of one's nature, without the baggage that comes along with an emotional attachment to someone. There is real pleasure experienced in these sorts of interactions. The reality is, however, that the men on my couch aren't glamorizing this. I was very conscious about not imposing my ideals about love onto my patients. They were the ones who would inevitably draw the conversation there, no matter what they initially came in for. I think that's because most sex is actually occurring in the context of a relationship, and therefore the relationship permeates the sex act. And even without the presence of a relationship, there are still human emotional needs beyond the carnal that intrude on sex—this is where it became most intriguing for me.

For my patients, sex had become love's surrogate. What they

couldn't get emotionally, what they didn't dare ask for, they sought through sex. Sex stood in for their ego strivings: their wish to be special, important, powerful, desired. Sex took the place of everything mother or wife or prostitute didn't provide. However, much of it was a substitute for what they couldn't summon from within. Instead of learning to care for themselves, they would turn to fantasy, creating scripts and looking for an actress to play a role. This role changes, too, according to what a man needs at the time. These guys hope that the women they're with can intuit what they want and become that for them. None of this has anything to do with the real woman.

This is not love, for the act, with all of its drama and intensity, is actually no deeper than the interaction you can have with the cashier at the 7-Eleven.

I once had a patient who was a very successful songwriter. In our first session he told me, "I write songs about love for a living, but I don't believe in love. I'm just doing it for money."

I thought it was very telling that this was the first statement he wanted to make. Of all he could have chosen to reveal about himself, this is what he wanted to lead with.

"It's all an illusion," he continued. "Pheromones, dopamine, everything boils down to sex. Procreation. Love is a romantic fantasy."

He couldn't have sounded more blasé.

"Do you wish love was real?" I asked.

"No, I want to live in reality."

"And reality is simply biology?"

"Well, okay. When people talk about being in love, what

they're really saying is 'This person makes me feel good about myself.' But it's just fucking validation. Don't get me wrong, I like validation. I live for it actually. But you never get it consistently; that's why I feel like shit right now. My ex-girlfriend sucks."

"So if it's all biology then let's just accept that. Celebrate that!"

He stood and walked around my office. "I need to move around," he said. "I hate this 'let's sit and psychobabble' stuff. Is this supposed to be helpful? I'm here to be helped." Then he sat again, but this time on the footstool by my feet, and just stared me down at close range, in silence, as if he was trying to read something about me. I stared back, my eyebrows raised, a little unnerved.

Then he abruptly got up and started pacing again.

"You're easy on the eyes, you know that?"

"You're getting distracted," I said. "I thought you wanted to be helped."

"Sorry, I'm ADD and I had too much coffee. I don't know what I'm saying. I'm lost. I'm a mess."

"You're saying that love is all biology, and I'm saying, 'So what? Enjoy that then.'"

"No, that's fucking empty, man," he said, returning to the couch.

"Then what do you want?" I asked.

"I want it to *mean* something."

"Then let it mean something."

"But it's meaningless."

"I guess you're right. You're one existential mess!"

"If you're telling me to lay down the coffee and the Kierkegaard—sorry, honey, that's my world."

"Honey?"

"Sorry, sorry, Doctor!" he said, flashing a flirtatious smile.

We both laughed.

"Have you ever felt love?" I said.

"Yes. I guess. I thought I was in love with my ex. I had all of those feelings one thinks constitute love."

"So, some feelings *do* exist."

"I thought so. Probably just chemical reactions, though." He took his cell phone from his pocket and played with it.

"Did she disappoint you?"

"That's a fucking understatement."

"So she let you down, and now you dump on the whole idea of love. You discount *everything*?"

"If my manager calls, I need to take it," he said.

"Do you need to be loved?"

"Yeah."

Because most of us don't understand love, we don't know what to expect from it. I didn't yet know what had happened in his relationship, but he evidently had some expectations that had been dashed, which resulted in this philosophical attack. However, I knew that it's hard to deny the deep hunger we all have for what we call love. And I knew that the experience of yearning would be real for him. So what if biological imperatives and a need for validation are part of the process? He had missed the higher essence of love, the sum of its parts.

"Love is bigger than just romantic love between two people," I said. "It's expansive. You can love animals, nature, children, friends. We have an inborn need to give and receive, and we can do it in many ways beyond just being hung up on one person, one love object. You can love everything around you in some way."

He didn't respond with words, he simply looked incredulous, so I continued to make my case.

"Tell me something that you love."

"Playing guitar."

"What do you love about playing guitar?"

"I get lost in the sound. It's effortless."

"Don't put it into words. Think about it quietly."

"Okay . . ."

"Can you *feel* how you love it?"

"This is weird. What are you asking me to do?"

"Humor me."

He paused. "Okay. Yeah, I do feel a warmth."

"Now try to magnify that feeling."

"Uhhh . . . fine . . ."

"Now think of something else you love."

"My little sister."

"Sit with that. Let it build inside of you."

His eyes moistened.

"You just generated it. You can cultivate as much love as you want, anytime."

We went on for a while, and I learned of his love for many things, including his deceased dog Sherman and popsicles with cream in the middle. I felt uncomfortable because I could feel his condescension even as he tried to follow my directions. He definitely thought I was all Pollyanna about love. But he was also desperately unhappy enough to humor me. So we continued with the exercise over and over, naming many people and activities, and he *was* able to generate the sensation of love and sustain it, proving to him my point that the feeling of love could be cultivated. I wanted him to admit that at least that was real, concrete. He could trust that feeling in his body. And he did admit that it felt good.

We met only one more time, after which he dropped out of treatment abruptly to go on tour in Europe. In our final session, he came in talking about how he had to leave but wasn't excited because nothing excited him anymore. "The whole world is pointless." But maybe he'd come in looking for me to give him one flicker of hope before our time was over.

"Doc, can you just define love for me?"

I was on the spot and began to fumble for words. "Well, the love that we glamorize is a pleasurable, visceral sensation, but loving is actually a skill that includes a broad range of behaviors and feelings. . . ."

He held up his hands. "Doc, please stop. Really? Is that what you're going to tell people? I think you need to come up with something better than that. Something easier to remember, a little mantra, and please, less clinical-sounding!"

He was right. That did sound pretty boring.

"Fine, fine. Okay," I said. "Love is recognizing the beauty in everyone and everything around you—and you need love to find your inspiration again, to create, to write songs."

A month later I got an email from him, from Brussels. He thanked me. He also wrote, "I have one last question. What if I never find love again?"

I emailed back: "I trust that you will. If there's one thing I know for sure, it's that everyone needs love, both to give and receive it. This doesn't die when a relationship ends. Love is bigger than one person."

He also wrote that after thinking about our final conversation, he'd laid down the Sartre and picked up some Rumi.

To my great pleasure, this shift in thinking about love happened often. I actually had guys saying to me, "I'm not looking for love anymore. I want to be love." I often paused to marvel at this evolution from popular expressions such as "women are bitches" to "I used to wonder if I was loved. Now I ask if I ever loved." I couldn't believe men were using phrases like that with me. Their focus was shifting from what they could get to what they could provide, and I was well pleased.

Rami and I had been stable for some time, so we decided that this long-distance thing had to come to an end. If our relationship was ever going to work, one of us had to move. Then, in true Rami fashion, he showed up at my front door and announced, "I'm moving to New York." He had packed some of his belongings into his car and driven up from Florida. "You're the love of my life," he proclaimed. "I don't care what the cost, we are going to be together."

I was exultant. Finally, the tension over who would move would end and I would have both Rami and New York. I said good-bye to my roommates in Times Square and rented a place for the two of us on the Upper West Side. I saw him for dinner every day, and we would finally lie down together each night. This realization of my wishes, however, lasted approximately two months. I will spare you the details and just say that the rest pretty much went as follows: He bought an engagement ring. We fought. He returned the ring and bought himself a

Rolex. We fought. He threw the Rolex into the Hudson. He moved back to Florida.

I was alone in New York for the first time in my own apartment.

This wasn't a breakup, and there were no hard feelings either. We simply returned to our long-distance arrangement. Rami missed his big house in Florida; he said he couldn't live the way people do in Manhattan.

I thought about what he'd said as I lay in my studio apartment, a space so tight that I could reach out and open my refrigerator door from my bed. I realized that I could use an upgrade in my own standard of living; how long was I going to live with a kitchen the size of a phone booth and mice skittering around as I slept? (I kept my keys and shoes nearby to throw at them in the middle of the night.)

Then I remembered my promise to move back to Florida after one year in New York—and the real reason I wouldn't go back. We had trust issues. I hadn't felt safe, so I wasn't prepared to take the risk. Instead I had decided to stay in New York, rather than face my anxiety about moving in with Rami. This is crazy, I thought. I had challenged my clients to be bold and courageous about the ones they love. I decided it was time for me to take a risk.

So I finally called Rami and told him that I would be moving to Florida. I sold my practice, sublet my apartment, told all of my friends good-bye.

"Are you crazy?" they asked when I gathered them at an Upper West Side wine bar to make my announcement. Despite their consternation, I felt very peaceful, the kind of calm you feel when you get off the fence and finally make a decision. Rami and I were both excitedly making plans for our new life together.

A few days later, as I was packing, Rami called.

"Maybe it would be better if you got your own place down here instead of moving in with me," he suggested.

"What? Why?"

"What if we get bored of each other?" he said. "I don't want to feel trapped." He continued with a jumble of words and phrases that barely made sense, but sounded like bad excuses. I was so overwhelmed, I could barely hear.

"Maybe I should have you sign some paperwork that says I'm not financially responsible for you," he muttered.

I dropped the phone, fell to the floor of my packed-up studio, and wailed.

Rami had balked, just like Mohinder the cabdriver had said he would if I ever made myself truly available to him.

I had believed that if only I took the leap we would find stability. I realized that by withholding myself all these years, I had maintained just enough distance for Rami to be comfortable—even though he always blamed *me* for being away.

Then it hit me. Oh my God. My practice! I had just signed it over to a new owner. I also had to be out of my apartment in two weeks. I had just changed my entire life for what I believed to be a bold decision about love.

I collected myself and booked an immediate flight to a place I'd always wanted to go: California. In a matter of days, I had sublet a room in a beautiful house across from the beach, and I flew back to New York to pack the last of my things. I decided to put it all in brown cardboard boxes and mail everything to myself. As I was addressing the boxes to San Diego, I wasn't surprised when

Rami showed up at my door, wanting to talk. This time, I simply asked him to drop the boxes off at the post office for me. They were too heavy, I said.

And that was it.

Yes, I was hurt by Rami. The lies, the womanizing, the rejection. However, I'll never believe I was a fool for the decision I made to move or my decision to love this man. For my loyalty is to the integrity of love itself. Yes, he let me down, but that was due to his own struggle with loving. I am proud of my bravery and my commitment to loving, and even though I often don't get it right, each time I practice, it takes me to a higher place.

One of the most common questions that patients—both men and women who've been felled by heartbreak—ask is this: Why do it again? Why should I open up? These people are trying to reconcile the fact that the possibility of getting scourged by love always exists, yet they still need it. But giving in to the fear and rejecting relationships doesn't protect them, because the alternative is to end up lonely and still suffer pain. So I answer honestly: Yes, you will get hurt, and that's why one of the most important lessons in love is being able to accept that pain is part of the process—though there is beauty in all of the toughest of emotions about love.

I couldn't become jaded or cynical; that would never be my style. I didn't lose my preference for romance; rather I added a richer and more realistic perspective as a result of my work with men. Each time I concluded that Rami was a certain villain, he showed me his tremendous capacity for goodness. That dichotomy busied my mind for a long time, until I realized that it's not actually confusing, it's just human nature. This realization was liberating and helped take me to a place beyond judgment. I may have had to break up with him ten times, but going through that process was similar to my challenge to face the truths of my male clients. I had to overcome the insecurities they roused in me, to get to a place of compassion and understanding.

It took me a long time and hard work, but these guys taught me to be patient, brave, and tolerant. I never thought any of these virtues to be as dazzling or enchanting as my beloved romantic infatuations, but they are the pillars that provide the foundation that allows the fun parts of love to endure. I started out unable to answer men's questions about the nature of love, but through my connection with each of them, we were able to define a love that was ultimately healing for both patient and doctor.

POSTSCRIPT

Rami returned to his beloved single life and to traveling, though now he builds orphanages in developing countries.

I have a private practice in Los Angeles and am happily married to a man who has brought me more adventure than my fantastical imagination could ever have conjured. He is from Iowa.

ACKNOWLEDGMENTS

BRANDY:

The idea for this book was conceived on a solo drive from Los Angeles to a small town in the desert the Christmas following my recent arrival from New York. The stark landscape always calms my mind, and the ideas for this book emerged so quickly that I pulled over and wrote my outline in a Walgreens parking lot. I want to thank Sue Schrader and Matt Johnston, my first friends in California, who after reading that outline encouraged me to follow through and write the book. Their belief in what I had to say played a large role in propelling me forward. Thank you.

I also want to give a heartfelt thanks to Rami, whose name I have changed here because he did not ask to have the details of our relationship made public. Further, the book is clearly written from my point of view. However, I called him on several occasions asking for his consent to tell each and every Rami story. His only response:

"Make sure that you write that I still love you." My reply: "Seriously, this book is going to be published!" He remained typically magnanimous in spirit, saying that he supported the book and me telling my truth. But he always added, "Just make sure the reader knows how much I love you." I hope that despite revealing the most harrowing parts of our relationship, his wish has been granted.

I also would like to express my gratitude to David Rensin. It has been a real honor as a first-time author to work with an acclaimed professional. He took on a risky project with an unknown author because, as he often said, he believed in the material. I am deeply grateful that he made that choice. I am also grateful for his interest in the psychology of sex, his steadfast reverence for the patients represented in this book, and his ability to humanize their struggles. David was also a nurturing and patient guide who allowed me the space to amble through learning the craft of writing. He had an uncanny ability to get me to open up. I was originally resistant to sharing my personal story, but he prodded, coaxed, seduced, and beguiled until I allowed the woman to emerge from behind the professional façade. And he was there every step of the way to support me through my anxieties about telling the truth about my anxieties. He pushed me to be vulnerable and authentic, just as I had pushed my patients.

To my literary agent, Brian DeFiore, thank you for your unwavering belief in this book through thick and thin, and to Denise Silvestro of Berkley Books, thank you for taking a chance on me.

Thank you to Suzie Peterson, Amy Alkon, and Stephanie Willen for thoughtful reads and edits.

Brian Pike of Creative Artists Agency: I appreciate your enthusiastic interest in the book and your authentic vision for a television series based on the material.

Thank you to my dear girlfriends who supported this project.

Suzy Coyle, a voice of wisdom and insight. Karen Sandoval for telling me that my vulnerability is not embarrassing, it's beautiful. To Amy Reichenbach, a constant source of humor, challenge, and inspiration. Other friends who offered support and encouragement: Beth and Laura Reichenbach, Wendy McCarty, Mary Van Lent, Steve Smith, Robert Slusarenko, Jamie Cook-Tate.

To my patients, those written about and not, thank you for the honor of allowing me to be a part of your journey. Your participation in my learning process will continue to pay forward, as my future patients will be in better hands because of you.

To my mother, Irene Dunn: I have been well loved by you, and thus my ability to love has become a powerful tool for the healing of others. Thanks to Robert Dunn, Brian Dunn, and Carla Spooner for the humorous insights they added.

Finally, love and thanks to Francis Engler, my husband. On the day of that lonely drive to the desert, I had declined to travel with you, a fateful decision that led to our separation for two long years. I decided to write this book to fill my time and ward off the pain of missing you. Your relentless support of my decision to write the book, and your unshakeable confidence that I could do it, filled and inspired me. The lessons I learned in this book, and the questions I asked about love, have all led me to you.

DAVID:

Many thanks to Brian DeFiore, whose faith from the outset in my enthusiasm for bringing Brandy aboard and working with her to create this unusual book was matched only by his steadfast guidance to see it through.

For moral support, friendship, good cheer, and listening to me ramble on about this book for two years—even if some had to fortify themselves with drink—thank you to Cynthia Price, Amy Alkon (for more than she realizes), Nancy Rommelmann, Lisa Kusel, Zorianna Kit, Sara Grace, Erika Schickel, Steve Randall, Jane Ayer, Joseph Mailander, Lisa Strum Sweetingham, Greg Critser, Eric Estrin, Bill Zehme, Denise Silvestro and her excellent team at Berkley, Judd Klinger, Roman Genn, Joe Rensin, Jill Stewart, Jane and Gary Peterson, Paul Peterson, George and Charlotte Clinton, Gravtee, SA Jennifer Laurie (always), Steve Oney, and Francis Engler. If I forgot to mention anyone, it was accidental, and probably because I don't get enough sleep.

I'm most grateful and indebted to Dr. Brandy Engler for trusting me to be a partner. She fearlessly stepped up and shared her own life and loves to give this book unique dimension. She also cheerfully indulged my insatiable curiosity and relentless passion for veering off the track into meandering philosophical discussions about the psychology of sex, love, and relationships—*when we were supposed to be working.* I confess I wanted to hear what she thought about what I thought, and I shamelessly plundered her expertise. What I got from Brandy was a nonjudgmental, challenging, and consistently refreshing point of view. All of it went into the book, so I guess we were working after all.

I recommend that you sit on her couch.

Finally, as always, my love and gratitude for my wife, Suzie Peterson, and son, Emmett Rensin. Their grace in life is my earthly reward. People may tell me everything, but you both mean everything to me.